IMPROVING MEDICAL EDUCATION

Enhancing the Behavioral and Social Science Content of Medical School Curricula

Committee on Behavioral and Social Sciences in
Medical School Curricula

Board on Neuroscience and Behavioral Health

Patricia A. Cuff and Neal A. Vanselow, *Editors*

INSTITUTE OF MEDICINE
OF THE NATIONAL ACADEMIES

THE NATIONAL ACADEMIES PRESS
Washington, D.C.
www.nap

D1415962

THE NATIONAL ACADEMIES PRESS 500 Fifth Street, N.W. Washington, DC 20001

NOTICE: The project that is the subject of this report was approved by the Governing Board of the National Research Council, whose members are drawn from the councils of the National Academy of Sciences, the National Academy of Engineering, and the Institute of Medicine. The members of the committee responsible for the report were chosen for their special competences and with regard for appropriate balance.

This study was supported by Award No. N01-OD-4-2139, Task Order No. 112, and Grant No. 046078 between the National Academy of Sciences and the National Institutes of Health, Office of Behavioral and Social Science Research and The Robert Wood Johnson Foundation. Any opinions, findings, conclusions, or recommendations expressed in this publication are those of the author(s) and do not necessarily reflect the view of the organizations or agencies that provided support for this project.

International Standard Book Number 0-309-09142-X (Book)
International Standard Book Number 0-309-53001-6 (PDF)
Library of Congress Control Number: 2004105404

Additional copies of this report are available from the National Academies Press, 500 Fifth Street, N.W., Lockbox 285, Washington, DC 20055; (800) 624-6242 or (202) 334-3313 (in the Washington metropolitan area); Internet, http://www.nap.edu.

For more information about the Institute of Medicine, visit the IOM home page at: **www.iom.edu.**

The serpent has been a symbol of long life, healing, and knowledge among almost all cultures and religions since the beginning of recorded history. The serpent adopted as a logotype by the Institute of Medicine is a relief carving from ancient Greece, now held by the Staatliche Museen in Berlin.

*"Knowing is not enough; we must apply.
Willing is not enough; we must do."*
—Goethe

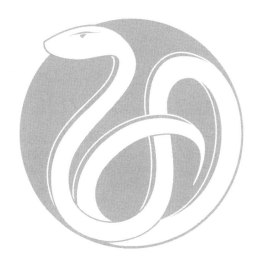

INSTITUTE OF MEDICINE
OF THE NATIONAL ACADEMIES

Adviser to the Nation to Improve Health

THE NATIONAL ACADEMIES
Advisers to the Nation on Science, Engineering, and Medicine

The **National Academy of Sciences** is a private, nonprofit, self-perpetuating society of distinguished scholars engaged in scientific and engineering research, dedicated to the furtherance of science and technology and to their use for the general welfare. Upon the authority of the charter granted to it by the Congress in 1863, the Academy has a mandate that requires it to advise the federal government on scientific and technical matters. Dr. Bruce M. Alberts is president of the National Academy of Sciences.

The **National Academy of Engineering** was established in 1964, under the charter of the National Academy of Sciences, as a parallel organization of outstanding engineers. It is autonomous in its administration and in the selection of its members, sharing with the National Academy of Sciences the responsibility for advising the federal government. The National Academy of Engineering also sponsors engineering programs aimed at meeting national needs, encourages education and research, and recognizes the superior achievements of engineers. Dr. Wm. A. Wulf is president of the National Academy of Engineering.

The **Institute of Medicine** was established in 1970 by the National Academy of Sciences to secure the services of eminent members of appropriate professions in the examination of policy matters pertaining to the health of the public. The Institute acts under the responsibility given to the National Academy of Sciences by its congressional charter to be an adviser to the federal government and, upon its own initiative, to identify issues of medical care, research, and education. Dr. Harvey V. Fineberg is president of the Institute of Medicine.

The **National Research Council** was organized by the National Academy of Sciences in 1916 to associate the broad community of science and technology with the Academy's purposes of furthering knowledge and advising the federal government. Functioning in accordance with general policies determined by the Academy, the Council has become the principal operating agency of both the National Academy of Sciences and the National Academy of Engineering in providing services to the government, the public, and the scientific and engineering communities. The Council is administered jointly by both Academies and the Institute of Medicine. Dr. Bruce M. Alberts and Dr. Wm. A. Wulf are chair and vice chair, respectively, of the National Research Council.

www.national-academies.org

Independent Report Reviewers

This report has been reviewed in draft form by individuals chosen for their diverse perspectives and technical expertise, in accordance with procedures approved by the NRC's Report Review Committee. The purpose of this independent review is to provide candid and critical comments that will assist the institution in making its published report as sound as possible and to ensure that the report meets institutional standards for objectivity, evidence, and responsiveness to the study charge. The review comments and draft manuscript remain confidential to protect the integrity of the deliberative process. We wish to thank the following individuals for their review of this report:

David B. Abrams, Brown University
Nancy E. Adler, University of California, San Francisco
William Branch, Emory University
F. Daniel Duffy, American Board of Internal Medicine
Neil J. Elgee, The Ernest Becker Foundation of the University of Washington
Marti Grayson, New York Medical College
William M. McDonald, Wesley Woods Health Center of Emory Healthcare
Joseph P. Newhouse, Harvard University
Susan Scrimshaw, University of Illinois at Chicago
Lu Ann Wilkerson, University of California, Los Angeles

Although the reviewers listed above have provided many constructive comments and suggestions, they were not asked to endorse the report's conclusions or recommendations nor did they see the final draft of the report before its release.

The review of this report was overseen by **Charles E. Phelps,** Provost, University of Rochester, New York, appointed by the National Research Council and the Institute of Medicine, who was responsible for making certain that an independent examination of this report was carried out in accordance with institutional procedures and that all review comments were carefully considered. Responsibility for the final content of this report rests entirely with the authoring committee and the institution.

Preface

There are a number of compelling reasons for all physicians to possess knowledge and skill in the behavioral and social sciences. Perhaps most important is that roughly half of the causes of mortality in the United States are linked to social and behavioral factors. In addition, our nation's population is aging and becoming more culturally diverse. Both of these trends highlight the need for enhanced physician capabilities in the behavioral and social sciences. Knowledge from these disciplines helps physicians understand the role of stress in both their patients' and their own lives and provides them with coping strategies. Moreover, many believe that competence in these areas is an important element in promoting humane medical practice.

Cognizant of important new research findings in the behavioral and social sciences and believing that all medical students should receive up-to-date instruction in these disciplines, the Office of Behavioral and Social Science Research of the National Institutes of Health and The Robert Wood Johnson Foundation asked the Institute of Medicine to conduct a study to accomplish three purposes:

- Review the current approaches used by medical schools to incorporate the behavioral and social sciences into their curricula.
- Develop a list of prioritized topics from the behavioral and social sciences for possible future inclusion in those curricula.
- Consider the barriers to incorporation of behavioral and social science content into medical school curricula, and suggest strategies for overcoming these barriers.

The committee's ability to respond to the first part of its charge was made difficult by the lack of a comprehensive database on current behavioral and social science content and teaching techniques in medical school curricula and by a relatively sparse literature on behavioral and social science instruction in the medical school setting. As a result, the committee was forced to draw some of its conclusions from existing databases that were incomplete and from information obtained in its own survey of selected medical schools.

The committee regarded the development of a prioritized list of behavioral and social science topics for inclusion in medical school curricula as the most important part of its work. Reducing the list to a realistic size was a difficult process that required extensive discussion and debate. The committee believes, however, that its ultimate recommended list not only contains highly important topics but also is compact enough for inclusion in the tightly packed 4 years of the medical school curriculum. It should also be emphasized that the committee does not recommend a specific behavioral and social science curriculum. Instead, it has chosen to outline those topics to which it believes all medical students should be exposed and to make a few suggestions regarding teaching techniques that might be employed. The way in which this material is woven into a given curriculum should be decided by the medical school's curriculum committee and will almost certainly vary from school to school.

The committee also discovered that there is very little literature on either barriers to the inclusion of the behavioral and social sciences in medical school curricula or strategies that might be employed to overcome such barriers. This portion of the report is therefore based largely on literature related to medical school curriculum change in general and on the experience of committee members, several of whom have been intimately involved with curriculum revisions at their own institutions.

Two other important points should be emphasized. First, the committee recognizes that medical education is a continuum that begins in the prebaccalaureate years and continues through medical school, graduate medical education, and practice. It believes that material from the behavioral and social sciences should be incorporated into each of these phases but has restricted its recommendations to the 4 years of medical school in the belief that including other parts of the continuum would be going beyond its charge.

Second, the importance of an institutional commitment to behavioral and social science instruction cannot be overemphasized. Without a firm belief on the part of medical school faculty and administration that knowledge and skill in the behavioral and social sciences are an important part of a physician's education and training, the recommendations contained in this report will be ineffective in producing change.

It is difficult to capture in words the enthusiasm with which this report is submitted. All who participated in the study are convinced that knowledge and skill in the behavioral and social sciences are essential to good medical practice. The committee sincerely hopes that the conclusions and recommendations contained in this report will serve as a catalyst for the improvement of behavioral and social science education in U.S. medical schools.

Neal A. Vanselow, M.D., *Chair*
Committee on Behavioral and
Social Sciences in Medical
School Curricula

Acknowledgments

The committee recognizes the tremendous efforts of several individuals whose contributions invigorated meeting discussions and enhanced the quality of this report. For their expert advice, opinions, and willingness to assist, the committee thanks its consultants Michael G. Goldstein and Michael E. Whitcomb. The committee also acknowledges with appreciation the testimony of M. Brownell Anderson, DeWitt C. Baldwin, Jr., Barbara Barzansky, Gerry Dillon, Richard Holloway, Cathy Lazarus, and Lesly T. Mega. Additional thanks go to Robby Reynolds, Nielufar Varjavand, Brenda Butler, Jason Satterfield, Doug Post, and Alan Cross for their assistance to the committee in gathering data on specific topics. Special appreciation is extended to Janet Fleetwood, Gordon Harper, and Steven Locke for their extra efforts and repeated attention to the ongoing information and support needs of the study, and to Julian Bird, who spent many hours working on the domain material that served as the basis for the committee's Delphi process.

Lawrence J. Fine, M.D., Dr.P.H., and Raynard Kington, M.D., Ph.D., of the National Institutes of Health, Office of Behavioral and Social Sciences Research, and The Robert Wood Johnson Foundation deserve particular recognition for generously supporting the vision that medical education can be improved through the enhancement of behavioral and social science training of medical students in the United States.

The committee would be remiss if it did not also acknowledge the hard work and dedication of the study staff in the Board on Neuroscience and Behavioral Health. Andy Pope was a valuable resource with his extensive know-how as the board director, and Gooloo Wunderlich, with her strict attention to the evidence base, ensured that the most recent factual data would be considered. For initiating the study, the committee thanks former staff members Terry Pelmar, board director; Lauren Honess-Morreale, study director; Olufunmilola Odegbile, research assistant; and Allison Berger, project assistant. Special appreciation goes to Patricia Cuff, study director; Benjamin Hamlin, research assistant; and Judy Estep, senior project assistant for stepping in and bringing the study to its conclusion. Patricia did an excellent job of keeping the committee informed about the report's status during and after the period of transition; Ben stalwartly pursued the daunting task of verifying references; and Judy, with her word processing ability and experience, was instrumental in getting the report into production. Final thanks go to writing and editorial consultants Rona Briere, Kathi Hanna, and Michael Hayes.

Contents

EXECUTIVE SUMMARY   1
    Abstract, 1
    Role of Behavioral and Social Factors in Health and Disease, 2
    Why Physicians Need Education and Training in the
       Behavioral and Social Sciences, 4
    Statement of Task, 4
    Current State of the Behavioral and Social Sciences in
       Curricula of U.S. Medical Schools, 5
    Conclusions and Recommendations, 6

1   INTRODUCTION   15
    Role of Behavioral and Social Factors in Health and Disease, 15
    Purpose of the Study, 18
    Study Origin and Tasks and Organization of the Report, 18

2   CURRENT APPROACHES TO INCORPORATING THE
   BEHAVIORAL AND SOCIAL SCIENCES INTO
   MEDICAL SCHOOL CURRICULA   20
    Summary, 20
    The Behavioral and Social Sciences in Current Medical
       School Curricula, 22
    Barriers to Systematic Analysis of the Behavioral and
       Social Sciences in Medical School Curricula, 24
    Inventory of Current Behavioral and Social Science
       Content in Medical School Curricula, 27

Approaches of Selected Medical Schools to Integrating
   Behavioral and Social Science Content into Their
   Curricula, 32
Need for an Improved Database on the Status of Behavioral
   and Social Science Instruction in U.S. Medical Schools, 50

3 THE BEHAVIORAL AND SOCIAL SCIENCES IN
   MEDICAL SCHOOL CURRICULA   52
   Summary, 52
   Mind–Body Interactions in Health and Disease, 58
   Patient Behavior, 63
   Physician Role and Behavior, 68
   Physician–Patient Interactions, 74
   Social and Cultural Issues in Health Care, 79
   Health Policy and Economics, 83

4 STRATEGIES FOR INCORPORATING THE BEHAVIORAL
   AND SOCIAL SCIENCES INTO MEDICAL SCHOOL
   CURRICULA   87
   Summary, 87
   Barriers to Incorporating the Behavioral and Social Sciences
      into Medical School Curricula, 89
   Strategies for Curriculum Change, 90

REFERENCES   99

APPENDIXES

A Methods   119
B Committee and Staff Biographies   135

INDEX   141

Tables, Figures, and Boxes

TABLES

ES-1   Behavioral and Social Science Topics of High and Medium Priority for Inclusion in Medical School Curricula, 10

2-1   Methods for Teaching Basic Communication Skills, 25

2-2a   Number of Hours Selected LCME Hot Topics Are Taught Throughout the 4 Years of Medical School, 28

2-2b   Percentage of Medical Schools Teaching Specific Topics During Each Year of Medical School, 29

2-2c   Medical Student Satisfaction with Selected Topics at Time of Graduation, 30

3-1   Behavioral and Social Science Topics of High and Medium Priority for Inclusion in Medical School Curricula, 56

FIGURES

1-1   Model of the determinants of health, 17

A-1   MEDLINE search results, 120

A-2   Results of electronic multiple-database search, 121

xvii

BOXES

2-1   Schools with Educational Programs in the Behavioral and Social
        Sciences, Based on the Literature and Website Information, 33
2-2   Behavioral and Social Science Education in the Medical School
        Curriculum of Ohio State University, 34
2-3   Behavioral and Social Science Education in the Medical School
        Curriculum of the University of California, San Francisco (UCSF), 36
2-4   Behavioral and Social Science Education in the Medical School
        Curriculum of the University of Rochester, 41
2-5   Behavioral and Social Science Education in the Medical School
        Curriculum of the University of North Carolina, 45

3-1   Complex Communication Skills, 77

A-1   List of Interested Associations, Organizations, and Medical Schools
        Represented by Invited Speakers, 122
A-2   Suggested Curriculum Content Organized by Five Domains, 124

IMPROVING MEDICAL EDUCATION

Executive Summary

ABSTRACT

In response to growing recognition of the role played by behavioral and social factors in health and disease, the National Institutes of Health and The Robert Wood Johnson Foundation asked the Institute of Medicine to conduct a study of medical school education in the behavioral and social sciences. The study included a review of the approaches used by medical schools to incorporate the behavioral and social sciences into their curricula, development of a prioritized list of behavioral and social science topics for future inclusion in those curricula, and an examination of ways in which barriers to the incorporation of behavioral and social science topics can be overcome.

The committee finds that existing databases provide inadequate information on behavioral and social science curriculum content, teaching techniques, and assessment methodologies in U.S. medical schools and recommends development of a new national behavioral and social science database. It also recommends that medical students be provided with an integrated behavioral and social science curriculum that extends throughout the 4 years of medical school. The committee identifies 26 topics in six behavioral and social science domains that it believes should be included in medical school curricula. The six domains are mind–body interactions in health and disease, patient behavior, physician role and behavior, physician–patient interactions, social and cultural issues in health care, and health policy and economics.

1

> *To help overcome multiple barriers to the incorporation of the behavioral and social sciences into medical school curricula, the committee recommends that the National Institutes of Health or private foundations establish behavioral and social sciences career development and curriculum development awards. Moreover, concerned that the U.S. Medical Licensing Examination currently places insufficient emphasis on test items related to the behavioral and social sciences, the committee recommends that the National Board of Medical Examiners ensure that the exam adequately covers the behavioral and social science subject matter recommended in this report.*

ROLE OF BEHAVIORAL AND SOCIAL FACTORS IN HEALTH AND DISEASE

For more than a decade it has been well established that approximately half of all causes of morbidity and mortality in the United States are linked to behavioral and social factors (McGinnis and Foege, 1993; NCHS, 2003a). In fact, the leading cause of preventable death and disease in the United States—smoking—significantly increases the risk of lung cancer and chronic lung disease, as well as the risk of heart disease and stroke (CDC, 1999; Mokdad et al., 2004; NCHS, 2003a). A sedentary lifestyle, along with poor dietary habits, has also been associated with increased risk of heart disease, as well as a myriad of other adverse health conditions, and may soon overtake tobacco as the leading cause of preventable death (Graves and Miller, 2003; Mokdad et al., 2004; Morsiani et al., 1985; U.S. DHHS, 2001). Alcohol consumption is the third leading cause of preventable death in the United States (Mokdad et al., 2004). And although moderate alcohol intake may have some protective effects against heart disease, excessive consumption has been linked to a variety of potentially preventable conditions (Maekawa et al., 2003; Nanchahal et al., 2000; Pessione et al., 2003).

Illnesses related to behavioral factors include, among others, cancer, heart disease, poor pregnancy outcome, chronic obstructive pulmonary disease, type II diabetes, and unintentional injury (Hoyert, 1996; NCHS, 2003a; NHLBI, 2003a,b; U.S. DHHS, 1996). In addition to these adverse health effects of harmful behaviors, psychological and social factors have been shown to influence chronic disease risk and recovery. Psychological factors, such as personality, developmental history, spiritual beliefs, expectations, fears, hopes, and past experiences, shape people's emotional reactions and behaviors regarding health and illness. Social factors, including support of family and friends, institutions, communities, culture, politics, and economics, can have profound effects as well. Indeed, scientific evidence is increasing on the effects of psychological and social factors on biology, and recent studies have demonstrated that psychosocial stress may be a significant risk factor for a variety of diseases (Barefoot et al., 2000; Carroll et al.,

1976; Everson et al., 1996; Frasure-Smith et al., 1993; Kawachi et al., 1996; Leserman et al., 2000; Mayne et al., 1996; Orth-Gomer et al., 1993). In the case of heart disease, for example, psychosocial stress appears to contribute directly to atherosclerotic processes by narrowing blood vessels, thus restricting circulation (Bairey Merz et al., 2002; Williams et al., 1991).

Theories underlying behavioral interventions aimed at modifying disease course are based on the assumptions that behavioral and psychosocial influences on disease course are modifiable and that curtailing unhealthy practices will slow disease progression or minimize the recurrence of disease following treatment (IOM, 2000). Understanding that behavior can be changed and that proven methods are available to facilitate such change allows physicians to provide optimal interventions—behavioral and nonbehavioral—to improve the health of patients. Identifying personal, familial, social, and environmental factors that may affect a patient's health enables physicians to provide better, more patient-centered care (IOM, 2001a, 2003a). In addition, physicians must be able to recognize their own personal and social biases and perceptions to best serve the needs of their patients.

Although the scientific evidence linking biological, behavioral, psychological, and social variables to health, illness, and disease is impressive, the translation and incorporation of this knowledge into standard medical practice appear to have been less than successful. To make measurable improvements in the health of Americans, physicians must be equipped with the knowledge and skills from the behavioral and social sciences needed to recognize, understand, and effectively respond to patients as individuals, not just to their symptoms. Sobel (2000:393), an expert in mind–body health care, notes that "more and more studies point to simple, safe and relatively inexpensive interventions that can improve health outcomes and reduce the need for more expensive medical treatments. Far from a new miracle drug or medical technology, the treatment is simply the targeted use of mind–body and behavioral medicine interventions in a medical setting." Thus, physicians with an understanding of disease causation that extends beyond biomedical approaches are more likely to see better intervention outcomes than have been achieved to date (IOM, 2000).

A number of demographic factors in the United States also underscore the need for more attention to the behavioral and social components of health. First, the proportion of the population aged 65 and over is expected to grow by 57 percent by 2030 (U.S. Bureau of the Census, 1996), and with Americans now having an average life expectancy of 77 years (NCHS, 2003b), physicians need the knowledge and skills to care for this aging population. To this end, they must understand the interplay of social and behavioral factors (e.g., diet, exercise, and familial and social support) and the role these factors play in delaying or preventing the onset of disease and slowing its progression. Physicians also need to have been trained in pain management and means of improving quality-of-life measures that are essential to providing patient-centered care. Knowledge and skills in both of these areas are especially critical for the treatment of chronic conditions, common in this population, that require palliative care.

A second demographic change is the rising percentage of minorities in the overall U.S. population. According to U.S. census data, 26 percent of the current population is nonwhite, a proportion that is expected to increase to almost 47 percent by 2050 (U.S. Bureau of the Census, 1996). The country's growing cultural and ethnic diversity presents new challenges and opportunities for physicians and other health professionals, who must become culturally competent and better skilled in communicating and negotiating health management with diverse populations (Crawley et al., 2002; IOM, 2003c; Satterfield et al., 2004).

WHY PHYSICIANS NEED EDUCATION AND TRAINING IN THE BEHAVIORAL AND SOCIAL SCIENCES

It is clear that medical students with education in the behavioral and social sciences will be better equipped to recognize patients' risky behaviors and foster changes in those behaviors through appropriate interventions. Skills in the behavioral and social sciences are essential for the prevention of many chronic diseases and for the effective management of patients with these diseases. Communication skills, which are emphasized in the behavioral and social sciences, will assist physicians in building therapeutic relationships with their patients and increase the likelihood that patients will follow their advice. In addition, good communication skills and the cross-disciplinary education discussed in this report will improve their ability to relate to their colleagues in medicine, as well as other professionals.

Physicians truly wanting to influence patient behavior must also be aware of their patients' social contexts. Given the demographic trends noted above, this will inevitably translate into physicians encountering more elderly patients and those from a greater variety of cultures, who will need guidance in how best to utilize available therapeutic services within the changing health care system. These matters, too, are covered by a comprehensive behavioral and social science curriculum. Additionally, teaching medical students how to care for themselves, function in a team environment, use ethical judgment, and understand the usefulness of community resources can improve their job satisfaction and prevent burnout when they enter practice.

STATEMENT OF TASK

In this context, the Institute of Medicine convened the Committee on Behavioral and Social Sciences in Medical School Curricula to examine the content and effectiveness of behavioral and social science teaching in medical school education. The committee was asked to address the following charge:

1. Review the approaches used by medical schools that have tried to incorporate the behavioral and social sciences into their curricula.

2. Develop a list of prioritized topics from the behavioral and social sciences for possible inclusion in medical school curricula. As an alternative to a numerical list, clustered priorities (e.g., top, high, medium, and low) may be assigned to topic areas.

3. Provide options for how changes in curricula can be achieved, such as encouraging the leadership of medical schools to incorporate behavioral and social sciences, funding opportunities that would achieve this goal, or other novel approaches that would achieve this aim. In developing these options, the barriers to implementing curricula change and approaches to overcome these barriers should be considered.

The committee met five times between December 2002 and October 2003 and cast a broad net to capture the relevant information. It held public meetings with medical schools and other organizations to explore and discuss relevant information regarding the status of the teaching of the behavioral and social sciences in medical schools. The committee also reviewed and considered information from the published literature, medical school websites, and a variety of other sources. (See Appendix A for details regarding the methods used by the committee in conducting this study.)

CURRENT STATE OF THE BEHAVIORAL AND SOCIAL SCIENCES IN CURRICULA OF U.S. MEDICAL SCHOOLS

U.S. medical schools appear to be moving toward incorporating the behavioral and social sciences into their curricula in some way, and international efforts are under way to systematically include the behavioral and social sciences as part of the foundations of medical education (IIME, 2003). It is difficult to document with certainty, however, how much behavioral and social science is currently being taught in U.S. medical schools. This is the case because definitions of what constitutes the behavioral and social sciences vary, and difficulties abound in identifying medical school courses that include such components. For the purposes of this report, the behavioral and social sciences as applied to medicine are ideally defined as those research-based disciplines that provide physicians with empirically verifiable knowledge that serves as a foundation for understanding and influencing individual, group, and societal actions relevant to improving and maintaining health.

In reviewing the curricular content across U.S. medical schools, it became evident to the committee that there is significant variability in the teaching of the behavioral and social sciences: course titles differ; the number of hours of instruction varies; course content is inconsistent; the timing of instruction during the undergraduate experience differs (AAMC, 2003a; Milan et al., 1998; Muller,

1984); and whether or not the behavioral and social sciences are fully integrated[1] into students' 4-year education depends on the institution (Waldstein et al., 2001). A few medical schools do offer curricula in which behavioral and social science material is included in all 4 years of medical education, rather than being confined to the preclinical years. It appears more common, however, that behavioral and social science courses are taught during the first 2 years. In 2000, only 8 percent of the 62 U.S. medical schools that responded to a survey about their curricula reported that they had integrated programs of behavioral medicine that stressed the effects of human behavior on health and illness using a biopsychosocial model (Brook et al., 2000).

The Curriculum Management and Information Tool (CurrMIT) database of the Association of American Medical Colleges (AAMC) is the most comprehensive tool available for collecting and analyzing the content of medical school curricula. However, it is a voluntary system, and not all medical schools participate. It is designed to allow medical schools to examine the full spectrum of their curricula, track key trends, support innovations, and compare local curricula with those of other medical schools (AAMC, 1999a). Schools have flexibility regarding how they enter their data in the CurrMIT database, depending on program needs. As a result, data entry formats vary from school to school, as do the level of detail and the degree to which the information is updated. Currently, only 67 medical schools have entered course titles related to the behavioral and social sciences into the CurrMIT database (AAMC, personal communication, September 2003).

CONCLUSIONS AND RECOMMENDATIONS

In response to its charge, the committee developed several conclusions and recommendations aimed at enhancing the incorporation of the behavioral and social sciences into medical school curricula. These conclusions and recommendations, as well as strategies for accomplishing the specific tasks outlined in the committee's charge, are presented below.

Routine Survey of Behavioral and Social Science Curricula

The lack of national standardization among medical school curricula, of standardization in the terminology used to describe curricular content, and of a comprehensive strategy for creating a national database of medical school curricula makes it difficult to describe systematically the subject matter medical schools

---

[1]An integrated curriculum for the purposes of this report is one in which behavioral and social science subject matter is taught as part of other courses in the basic and clinical sciences, not as separate courses.

have incorporated into their curricula. The committee believes the creation of an improved, periodically updated database on the state of behavioral and social science instruction in U.S. medical schools would be of significant benefit to individual medical schools, credentialing bodies, government agencies, and professional organizations. An alternative to creating a new database would be to modify CurrMIT to produce these data. Because both are major undertakings, the decision to develop a new database or modify CurrMIT should be based on which method best collects behavioral and social science teaching information within the available resources. The committee also believes AAMC is the logical organization to design and operate such a database, as it has access to and is respected by all U.S. allopathic medical schools, and its staff has considerable experience and expertise in data collection and analysis. AAMC should consider collaborating with other relevant professional organizations, such as the American Association of Colleges of Osteopathic Medicine and the Liaison Committee on Medical Education (LCME), in the design and operation of the database.

It is beyond the scope of the committee's charge to specify the data that should be collected, the collection methodology, or the types of analyses that should be performed—matters that would best be decided by those using the database. It may be noted that the ad hoc survey conducted by the committee for this study reflects some of its thinking about the minimum contents of a curriculum database.

Conclusion 1. *Existing national databases provide inadequate information on behavioral and social science content, teaching techniques, and assessment methodologies. This lack of data impedes the ability to reach conclusions about the current state and adequacy of behavioral and social science instruction in U.S. medical schools.*

Recommendation 1: *Develop and maintain a database.* **The National Institutes of Health's Office of Behavioral and Social Sciences Research should contract with the Association of American Medical Colleges to develop and maintain a database on behavioral and social science curricular content, teaching techniques, and assessment methodologies in U.S. medical schools. This database should be updated on a regular basis.**

Behavioral and Social Science Content in Medical School Curricula

No physician's education would be complete without an understanding of the role played by behavioral and social factors in human health and disease, knowledge of the ways in which these factors can be modified, and an appreciation of how personal life experiences influence physician–patient relationships. The committee believes that each medical school should expect entering students to have completed course work in the behavioral and social sciences during their prebaccalaureate education and should inform prospective applicants of its behavioral and social science–related requirements and/or recommendations. Behavioral and social science instruction in medical school should build on this prebaccalaureate foundation. The committee also believes that material from the behavioral and social sciences should be included in the post–medical school phases of the medical education continuum. These phases include residency and fellowship training, as well as continuing (postgraduate) medical education. While the emphasis in this report is on the 4 years of medical school, the importance of continuing behavioral and social science education throughout a physician's career cannot be overemphasized.

This section presents the committee's response to the second part of its charge, to develop a list of prioritized topics from the behavioral and social sciences for possible inclusion in medical school curricula. The committee considers this to be the most important part of its work. The committee's recommended list of topics is supported by two conclusions reached during its deliberations.

> **Conclusion 2a.** *Human health and illness are influenced by multiple interacting biological, psychological, social, cultural, behavioral, and economic factors. The behavioral and social sciences have contributed a great deal of research-based knowledge in each of these areas that can inform physicians' approaches to prevention, diagnosis, and patient care.*

Some areas of the behavioral and social sciences have been more thoroughly researched and rigorously tested than others. This observation does not diminish the importance of those areas with less verifiable evidence, but rather points to the need for more research. One such example is the strong influence physicians' actions can have on the attitudes and values of medical students, even though this nonverbal form of communication has not been thoroughly tested (Ludmerer, 1999). In contrast, the importance of effective physician communication has received a fair amount of attention by researchers. The results of this research indicate that physicians need basic communication skills in order to take accurate patient histories, build therapeutic relationships, and engage patients in an educative process of shared decision making (IOM, 2001a, 2003a; Peterson et al., 1992; Safran et al., 1998).

> **Conclusion 2b.** *Within the clinical encounter, certain interactional competencies are critically related to the effectiveness and subsequent outcomes of health care. These competencies include the taking of the medical history, communication, counseling, and behavioral management.*

Providing the core content in the behavioral and social sciences identified in this report during the 4 years of medical school will introduce this material at a time when students perceive it to be most relevant and facilitate reinforcement of important concepts throughout the preclinical and clinical years. Moreover, integrating the curriculum so that behavioral and social science topics are included as part of other basic science and clinical courses, instead of being presented in separate courses, will enable the educational experience to simulate real-world experience, in which behavioral and social factors in health and disease must be considered in the context of complex clinical situations.

The committee recognizes that there are many important topics to which students must be exposed during their 4 years of medical school. As with any suggested change to medical school curricula, calls to include the behavioral and social sciences must be balanced against similar requests from other disciplines that are vying for precious teaching time. As noted earlier, however, evidence is mounting that tremendous strides could be made in preventing disease and promoting health if more attention were given to the behavioral and social science priorities outlined in this report. Knowing this, the committee selected potential priority topics on the basis of (1) relevant evidence-based articles and reports in the literature; (2) presentations to the committee by content experts and medical school representatives; (3) literature and other material from the AAMC and LCME; (4) considerations related to the health of the public, driven mainly by root causes of morbidity and mortality; and (5) the gap between what is known and what is actually done in practice.

Following extensive deliberations, a modified Delphi process was used to prioritize this initial list of topics. (A detailed description of this process is included in Appendix A.) Committee members rated each of the topics on the list using a scale system, and then assigned each high, medium, or low priority based on its mean score and standard deviation. This list was further refined and finalized using the collective and individual experience of the committee as experts in medical school curriculum development and reform in the behavioral and social sciences. The low priorities were then discarded, and the remaining 26 topics were categorized as top, high, or medium priority. The results of this process constitute the committee's recommendation for those behavioral and social science topics that should be included in medical school curricula. In the committee's view, the 20 topics ranked top and high must be included in medical school curricula and were therefore combined into one high-priority group. The 6 medium-priority topics are also important and would significantly enhance the education of medical students. Inclusion of the medium priorities, as well as the depth of teaching and evaluation, is dependent upon the needs of the individual medical school.

The final listing of topics, presented in Table ES-1, is organized so as to have meaning for medical school curriculum committees.

The 26 recommended topics fall into the following six general domains of knowledge:[2]

---

[2]The order in which the various domains are listed is random and does not reflect the committee's view of their relative importance.

TABLE ES-1 Behavioral and Social Science Topics of High and Medium Priority for Inclusion in Medical School Curricula

Domain	High Priority	Medium Priority
Mind–Body Interactions in Health and Disease	• Biological mediators between psychological and social factors and health • Psychological, social, and behavioral factors in chronic disease • Psychological and social aspects of human development that influence disease and illness • Psychosocial aspects of pain	• Psychosocial, biological, and management issues in somatization • Interaction among illness, family dynamics, and culture
Patient Behavior	• Health risk behaviors • Principles of behavior change • Impact of psychosocial stressors and psychiatric disorders on manifestations of other illnesses and on health behavior	
Physician Role and Behavior	• Ethical guidelines for professional behavior • Personal values, attitudes, and biases as they influence patient care • Physician well-being • Social accountability and responsibility • Work in health care teams and organizations • Use of and linkage with community resources to enhance patient care	
Physician–Patient Interactions	• Basic communication skills • Complex communication skills	• Context of patient's social and economic situation, capacity for self-care, and ability to participate in shared decision making • Management of difficult or problematic physician–patient interactions
Social and Cultural Issues in Health Care	• Impact of social inequalities in health care and the social factors that are determinants of health outcomes • Cultural competency	• Role of complementary and alternative medicine
Health Policy and Economics	• Overview of U.S. health care system • Economic incentives affecting patients' health-related behaviors • Costs, cost-effectiveness, and physician responses to financial incentives	• Variations in care

• *Mind–body interactions in health and disease*—focuses on the four primary pathways of disease (biological, behavioral, psychological, and social). Students need to recognize and understand the many complex interactions among these pathways that may be compromising a patient's physical and/or mental health.

• *Patient behavior*—centers on behavioral pathways to promoting health and preventing disease. Educating medical students about behaviors that pose a risk to health will better equip them to provide appropriate interventions and influence patient behavior.

• *Physician role and behavior*—emphasizes the physician's personal background and beliefs as they may affect patient care, as well as the physician's own well-being.

• *Physician–patient interactions*—focuses on the ability to communicate effectively, which, as noted above, is a critical component of the practice of medicine.

• *Social and cultural issues in health care*—addresses what physicians need to know and do to provide appropriate care to patients with differing social, cultural, and economic backgrounds.

• *Health policy and economics*—includes those topics to which medical students should be exposed to help them understand the health care system in which they will eventually practice (although additional material regarding the U.S. health care system should be presented in the residency years).

Recommendation 2. *Provide an integrated 4-year curriculum in the behavioral and social sciences.* **Medical students should be provided with an integrated curriculum in the behavioral and social sciences throughout the 4 years of medical school. At a minimum, this curriculum should include the high-priority items delineated in this report and summarized in Table ES-1. Medical students should demonstrate competency in the following domains:**

- **Mind–body interactions in health and disease**
- **Patient behavior**
- **Physician role and behavior**
- **Physician–patient interactions**
- **Social and cultural issues in health care**
- **Health policy and economics**

Strategies for Incorporating Behavioral and Social Sciences into the Medical School Curriculum

The committee found that many barriers exist to incorporating the behavioral and social sciences into medical school curricula. Incorporating this material is a special challenge because of the nature of the content, the lack of faculty members in these disciplines, the lower status accorded to these disciplines by some in the medical school community, the lack of departmental status for behavioral and social science faculty, and the limited leadership and financial resources available to support such efforts.

Curriculum change rarely occurs without a champion or leader pushing the agenda forward. A well-supported career development program in the behavioral and social sciences would free promising faculty members from competing responsibilities so they could develop leadership skills and work toward incorporating the behavioral and social sciences into medical school curricula. Individuals receiving career development awards could also serve as resources to assist other medical schools attempting to enhance their behavioral and social science curricula.

> **Conclusion 3.** *Instruction in the behavioral and social sciences suffers from a lack of qualified faculty, inadequate support and incentives for existing faculty, and the absence of career development programs in the behavioral and social sciences.*

> **Recommendation 3.** *Establish a career development award strategy.* **Because the provision of career development awards has been an effective strategy for improving instruction and research in other health-related areas, the Office of Behavioral and Social Sciences Research of the National Institutes of Health or private foundations, or both, should establish a career development awards program to produce leaders in the behavioral and social sciences in medical schools.**

In addition to career development awards designed to produce medical school leaders in the behavioral and social sciences, the committee believes there is a need for a program of curriculum development awards. One major purpose of these awards would be to fund the development of model behavioral and social science curricula that could be emulated at other schools. Another major purpose, of course, would be to improve the behavioral and social science curriculum at the school receiving the award. Specifically, the award would enable a medical school to develop more-effective teaching techniques and create better ways of assessing student performance in the behavioral and social sciences. Such awards could also provide funding for a broad-based program of faculty development in the behavioral and social sciences, including both basic science and clinical faculty members.

> **Conclusion 4.** *Financial support for efforts by U.S. medical schools to improve their curricular content, teaching methodologies, and assessment of student performance in the behavioral and social sciences is inadequate.*

ion **4.** *Establish curriculum development demonstration*
The National Institutes of Health or private foundations,
d establish a program that funds demonstration projects
and social science curriculum development at U.S. medical

ρρ6-
13

/hich can occur within a specific course or on a medical licens-
is a critical process for determining the extent to which medical
astered course objectives. Faculty should be provided with the
other resources required to develop effective methods for evalu-
mpetence in the behavioral and social sciences. Provision of these
resources ... d include instruction in the development of quality behavioral and
social science examination questions. Because medical faculty members create
the test items for the U.S. Medical Licensing Examination (USMLE), improving
their test-writing skills at the local level will also serve to improve the quality of
the behavioral and social science questions on the licensing exam.

The material covered on the USMLE signals to both teachers and students
what is considered important in the field of medicine and thus what should be
emphasized in medical school curricula (Elstein, 1993; Swanson et al., 1992).
Despite considerable effort, the committee was unable to determine the percentage of USMLE test questions currently devoted to the behavioral and social sciences. It is the impression of a number of informed individuals interviewed by the
committee, however, that the amount of test material devoted to the behavioral
and social sciences has decreased. Furthermore, it is the belief of this committee
that the behavioral and social sciences are underrepresented on the USMLE. The
committee does not believe it is necessary to specify a particular number of behavioral and social science questions that should be on the exam. Rather, the
designed questions, however many it may take, should sufficiently cover the topics delineated in this report. Likewise, the committee believes the behavioral and
social sciences should be part of the new clinical skills exam that will soon be
included as part of the USMLE series.

Conclusion 5. *The subject matter covered by questions on the U.S. Medical
Licensing Examination has a significant impact on the curricular decisions
made by U.S. medical schools. The committee believes that the U.S. Medical
Licensing Examination currently places insufficient emphasis on test items
related to the behavioral and social sciences.*

Recommendation 5. *Increase behavioral and social science content on the
U.S. Medical Licensing Examination.* **The National Board of Medical
Examiners should review the test items included on the U.S. Medical
Licensing Examination to ensure that it adequately reflects the topics in
the behavioral and social sciences recommended in this report.**

1

Introduction

ROLE OF BEHAVIORAL AND SOCIAL FACTORS IN HEALTH AND DISEASE

For more than a decade it has been well established that approximately half of all causes of morbidity and mortality in the United States are linked to behavioral and social factors (McGinnis and Foege, 1993; NCHS, 2003a). In fact, the leading cause of preventable death and disease in the United States—smoking— significantly increases the risk of lung cancer and chronic lung disease, as well as the risk of heart disease and stroke (CDC, 1999; Mokdad et al., 2004; NCHS, 2003a). A sedentary lifestyle, along with poor dietary habits, has also been associated with increased risk of heart disease, as well as a myriad of other adverse health conditions, and may soon overtake tobacco as the leading cause of preventable death (Graves and Miller, 2003; Mokdad et al., 2004; Morsiani et al., 1985; U.S. DHHS, 2001). Alcohol consumption is the third leading cause of preventable death in the United States (Mokdad et al., 2004). And although moderate alcohol intake may have some protective effects against heart disease, excessive consumption has been linked to a variety of potentially preventable conditions (Maekawa et al., 2003; Nanchahal et al., 2000; Pessione et al., 2003).

Illnesses related to behavioral factors include, among others, cancer, heart disease, poor pregnancy outcome, chronic obstructive pulmonary disease, type II diabetes, and unintentional injury (Hoyert, 1996; NCHS, 2003a; NHLBI, 2003a,b; U.S. DHHS, 1996). In addition to these adverse health effects of harmful behaviors, psychological and social factors have been shown to influence chronic disease risk and recovery. Psychological factors, such as personality, developmental history, spiritual beliefs, expectations, fears, hopes, and past experiences, shape people's emotional reactions and behaviors regarding health and illness. Social factors, including support of family and friends, institutions, communities, culture, politics, and economics, can have profound effects as well. Indeed, scientific evidence is increasing on the effects of psychological and social factors on biology, and recent studies have demonstrated that psychosocial stress may be a significant risk factor for a variety of diseases (Barefoot et al., 2000; Carroll et al., 1976; Everson et al., 1996; Frasure-Smith et al., 1993; Kawachi et al., 1996; Leserman et al., 2000; Mayne et al., 1996; Orth-Gomer et al., 1993). In the case of heart disease, for example, psychosocial stress appears to contribute directly to atherosclerotic processes by narrowing blood vessels, thus restricting circulation (Bairey Merz et al., 2002; Williams et al., 1991).

Theories underlying behavioral interventions aimed at modifying disease course are based on the assumptions that behavioral and psychosocial influences on disease course are modifiable and that curtailing unhealthy practices will slow disease progression or minimize the recurrence of disease following treatment (IOM, 2000). Understanding that behavior can be changed and that proven methods are available to facilitate such change allows physicians to provide optimal interventions—behavioral and nonbehavioral—to improve the health of patients. Identifying personal, familial, social, and environmental factors that may affect a patient's health enables physicians to provide better, more patient-centered care (IOM, 2001a, 2003a). In addition, physicians must be able to recognize their own personal and social biases and perceptions to best serve the needs of their patients.

Although the scientific evidence linking biological, behavioral, psychological, and social variables to health, illness, and disease is impressive, the translation and incorporation of this knowledge into standard medical practice appear to have been less than successful. To make measurable improvements in the health of Americans, physicians must be equipped with the knowledge and skills from the behavioral and social sciences needed to recognize, understand, and effectively respond to patients as individuals, not just to their symptoms. Sobel (2000:393), an expert in mind–body health care, notes that "more and more studies point to simple, safe and relatively inexpensive interventions that can improve health outcomes and reduce the need for more expensive medical treatments. Far from a new miracle drug or medical technology, the treatment is simply the targeted use of mind–body and behavioral medicine interventions in a medical setting." Thus, physicians with an understanding of disease causation that extends beyond biomedical approaches are more likely to see better intervention outcomes than have been achieved to date (IOM, 2000).

The limitations of a strictly biomedical approach to health care as described by Engle suggest the need for a model of medical school education designed to provide an integrative and multilevel understanding of how biological, psychological, and social variables interact in health and illness (Engel, 1977). Others have expanded upon and explicated such a biopsychosocial model (Anderson and

Scott, 1999; Evans and Stoddart, 1990). The term "biopsychosocial," however, appears to imply three separate spheres while omitting other key disciplines, such as the behavioral sciences and economics. A unified approach that is more inclusive than both the biomedical and biopsychosocial models is needed as a curricular framework for medical education (see Figure 1-1 for an example of such a model).

A number of demographic factors in the United States also underscore the need for more attention to the behavioral and social components of health. First, the proportion of the population aged 65 and over is expected to grow by 57 percent by 2030 (U.S. Bureau of the Census, 1996), and with Americans now having an average life expectancy of 77 years (NCHS, 2003b), physicians need the knowledge and skills to care for this aging population. To this end, they must understand the interplay of social and behavioral factors (e.g., diet, exercise, and familial and social support) and the role these factors play in delaying or preventing the onset of disease and slowing its progression. Physicians also need to have been trained in pain management and means of improving quality-of-life measures that are essential to providing patient-centered care. Knowledge and skills in both of these areas are especially critical for the treatment of chronic conditions, common in this population, that require palliative care.

A second demographic change is the rising percentage of minorities in the overall U.S. population. According to U.S. census data, 26 percent of the current

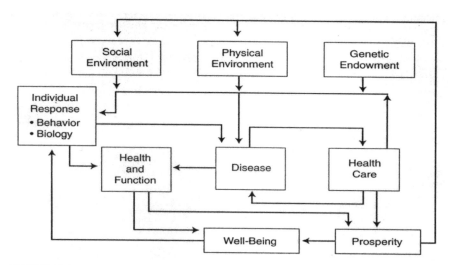

FIGURE 1-1 Model of the determinants of health. This model is a theoretical delineation of the interacting forces that contribute to the health, functional status, and well-being of an individual (or a population). Reproduced with permission from Elsevier Science Ltd. SOURCE: Evans and Stoddart (1990).

population is nonwhite, a proportion that is expected to increase to almost 47 percent by 2050 (U.S. Bureau of the Census, 1996). The country's growing cultural and ethnic diversity presents new challenges and opportunities for physicians and other health professionals, who must become culturally competent and better skilled in communicating and negotiating health management with diverse populations (Crawley et al., 2002; IOM, 2003c; Satterfield et al., 2004).

PURPOSE OF THE STUDY

For nearly three decades, persistent calls have been made to formally educate undergraduate medical students in the behavioral and social sciences to help establish a critical foundation for providing good clinical care (Bolman, 1995; Carr, 1998; Engel, 1977; Krantz et al., 1999). Increasingly, medical schools have introduced courses with behavioral and social science content into their curricula. However, current educational practices are uneven in their comprehensiveness and clinical applicability, and all too often, newly trained physicians cannot effectively translate behavioral and social science knowledge, skills, and attitudes into effective patient care. Given that nearly half of all patients present with conditions that are significantly influenced by such factors, continued lack of attention to this aspect of medical school training is no longer acceptable. Applying the behavioral and social sciences to medicine should not be a marginal effort, but a part of mainstream medical education.

STUDY ORIGIN AND TASKS AND
ORGANIZATION OF THE REPORT

This study was undertaken to enhance the behavioral and social sciences in medical school curricula in response to a request from the National Institutes of Health (NIH) and The Robert Wood Johnson Foundation. In the fall of 2002, the Institute of Medicine convened a committee to examine the content and effectiveness of behavioral and social science teaching in medical school education. The committee was asked to:

1. Review the approaches used by medical schools that have tried to incorporate behavioral and social sciences into their curricula.
2. Develop a list of prioritized topics from the behavioral and social sciences for possible inclusion in medical school curricula. As an alternative to a numerical list, clustered priorities (e.g., top, high, medium, and low) may be assigned to topic areas.
3. Provide options for how changes in curricula can be achieved, such as encouraging the leadership of medical schools to incorporate behavioral and social sciences, funding opportunities that would achieve this goal, or other novel approaches that would achieve this aim. In developing these options, the barriers

to implementing curricula change and approaches to overcoming these barriers should be considered.

To address the tasks described above, the committee met five times between December 2002 and October 2003, and cast a broad net to capture the relevant information. It held public meetings with medical schools and other organizations to explore and discuss relevant information regarding the status of teaching behavioral and social science in medical schools. The committee also reviewed and considered information from the published literature, medical school websites, and a variety of other sources. (See Appendix A for details regarding the methods that the committee used to address the statement of task.)

Each chapter of this report responds to one of the three tasks listed above. Chapter 2 reviews and describes currently available information on the incorporation of the behavioral and social sciences into undergraduate medical education. Included is a brief historical overview of curriculum changes in medical schools. Chapter 3 expands on the importance of including the behavioral and social sciences in medical school curricula. It also presents the 26 priority topics identified by the committee, along with the rationale for their selection. Included as well is a description of the type of content that would enable medical students to demonstrate competency in these areas. Chapter 4 provides an overview of successful strategies for creating and sustaining curriculum change in multiple areas of medical education. These strategies are discussed as they apply to behavioral and social science content and are accompanied by an analysis of the influence of national examinations on curricular content.

2

Current Approaches to Incorporating the Behavioral and Social Sciences into Medical School Curricula

TASK 1: *Review the approaches used by medical schools that have incorporated behavioral and social sciences into their curricula.*

SUMMARY: *Given the shifts in the structure of medical education that have occurred over time, increasing emphasis is now being placed on trying to educate students in the behavioral and social sciences throughout the 4 years of medical school using an integrated curriculum. Although only a small number of schools have accomplished this, content in the behavioral and social sciences does appear to be increasing in the curricula of many medical schools. This increase may be due in part to the requirement of the Liaison Committee on Medical Education (LCME) that, to be accredited, schools must include behavioral and socioeconomic subjects in their curricula.*

Because LCME does not specify how schools should incorporate any subjects, each school covers behavioral and social science content in a distinct manner appropriate to that institution. Each has its own course titles, materials, and content as well as teaching methods, often using a variety of faculty who may or may not be trained in the behavioral and social sciences. As a result, it is difficult if not impossible to specify the topics within the behavioral and social sciences that are being covered by all 126 U.S. medical schools without having a comprehensive, updated database. Such a database would allow individual medical schools to compare their curricula and student evaluation methods with those of other institutions that have successfully incorporated the behavioral and social sciences into their curricula. Other agencies and organizations concerned about ensuring that appropriate behavioral and social science information is being adequately taught to all U.S. medical students would also find this database useful. Based on the finding that existing national databases provide inadequate information on behavioral and social science content, teaching techniques, and assessment methodologies, the committee recommends the development of a comprehensive database that is updated on a regular basis.

The current structure of American medical education was adopted in the early 1900s and has not varied greatly since that time (Ludmerer, 1985). The basic sciences—anatomy, physiology, biochemistry, and microbiology—were introduced as a scientific foundation on which clinical practice knowledge and skills were built. In addition, the introduction of clinical science in the context of a university constituted a significant shift from a community practice–based, apprenticeship model of preparation for careers in medicine to one in which clinical medicine was taught by full-time faculty in a university-owned or university-affiliated teaching hospital. The Carnegie Foundation was instrumental in this reform of medical education, sponsoring a study by Abraham Flexner that became a blueprint for the transformation of medical schools nationally (Flexner, 1910). Over the years, however, shifts have occurred within the basic structure of medical education, including those related to learning techniques. An example is the movement from a focus on passive learning through lectures to active learning through the use of small-group exercises focused on cases and exercises that help integrate biological, psychological, and sociological perspectives, as well as clinical and basic science knowledge (Irby and Hekelman, 1997).

These new directions have coincided with significant changes in the practice of medicine and important developments in medicine itself. For example, medical schools have become only one element of academic health centers, which combine schools of various health professions, medical centers and hospitals, major clinical practice facilities, and research facilities. The practice of medicine itself has become highly organized and has generally moved from solo, private practices to practices in large groups and institutions. In addition, dramatic improvements have occurred in medical therapeutics, especially compared with the therapeutic modalities available a century ago, when it has been asserted that no more than six useful drugs were available (Osler and Harvey, 1976).

Another change is one that complicates attempts to identify and assess specific content taught in medical school courses. In the early 1900s, it was relatively easy to identify the science content (at least by subject area) of medical school courses because the courses were often given titles derived from the science being taught. Today, however, although the science content is still present, it is diffused across courses and is difficult to identify from outside the classroom and from a course title alone. For example, gross anatomy, which was classically taught through the dissection of a cadaver, may have given way to prosected demonstrations, "dissections" of a virtual human body in software programs, and a course on biological structure. Likewise, a course such as systemic function can include content ranging from cell biology to doctor–patient relationships (NCME, 2003).

Exploring the content of medical school curricula on the basis of course titles today is thus truly seeing through a glass darkly. This common disconnect between content and title can make the identification and assessment of the behavioral and social science content of medical coursework especially challenging, particularly when course titles are the only available source of data.

This chapter first outlines issues related to behavioral and social science content in medical school curricula, how these disciplines are integrated into the curriculum,[1] and the teaching methods that are generally used. It then identifies the barriers that hinder efforts to inventory behavioral and social science content in current medical school curricula. The third section presents the results of the committee's inventory efforts. The final section offers the committee's argument for the need to develop an improved database on the status of behavioral and social science instruction in U.S. medical schools and a recommendation to that end.

THE BEHAVIORAL AND SOCIAL SCIENCES IN CURRENT MEDICAL SCHOOL CURRICULA

The multidisciplinary perspective that emerges from studying the behavioral and social sciences provides students with an understanding of the patient as part of a broader social and environmental context that influences—and is influenced by—biological processes to produce health and illness behaviors, resilience, and functional capacity. Because the expression of human behavior occurs at the interface between the internal (physiological) and external (sociocultural) environments, and because some change in behavior is usually involved in biological and social dysfunction, the teaching of behavioral and social science is an effective way to integrate the various disciplinary perspectives in medicine (IOM, 1983). Given the breadth and diversity of the content of the behavioral and social sciences, however, it has been difficult for medical schools and medical school educators to agree on what constitutes the crucial core of behavioral and social science knowledge to which medical students should be exposed during their undergraduate education. Additionally, as the content encompassed by the behavioral and social sciences has grown, so, too, has the range of subject matter that could be taught to medical students.

---

[1]An integrated curriculum for the purposes of this report means that behavioral and social science subject matter is taught as part of other courses in the basic and clinical sciences, not as a separate course.

Some of the areas emphasized in instruction in the behavioral and social sciences in medical education have been driven by population health needs and risks. Given the strong interactions between behavioral factors and the etiology and pathogenesis of illness and disease (see Chapter 1), many schools opt to focus on specific biopsychosocial aspects of health and disease that affect populations. For example, substance abuse became the focus of a curriculum with behavioral and social science content for four medical schools in North Carolina because of the large and growing problems of substance abuse nationwide (Fang et al., 1998).

Some behavioral and social science content has already been considered part of classical medical education, serving to enlarge the content of courses in such areas as medical interviewing and the introduction to clinical medicine. Because effective communication skills are important to all physicians, the vast majority of schools teach such skills at some point within their curricula (AAMC, 1999b; Dube et al., 2000). Nevertheless, certain communication skills—such as communicating with diverse populations (in terms of culture, age, gender, and race), building trust in the presence of perceived or actual conflicts of interest, telecommunication, and physician–patient communication—are now receiving increased emphasis. As one example, the Macy Initiative in Health Communication at the University of Massachusetts Medical School was a curriculum designed to develop students' skills in delivering bad news to parents regarding their fetus or child, with a particular focus on communicating in the areas of genetic counseling, risk assessment, and birth defects (Pettus, 2002). Communication among physicians and other members of the health care team has also received attention in the curriculum, especially given the movement toward more-integrated health care systems.

The curricula in even traditional medical disciplines, such as psychiatry, have seen an expansion of behavioral and social science content. Although all schools of medicine have curricula in psychiatry, some focus on the overlap between mental and somatic health, or psychosomatic medicine, as many patients have significant emotional or behavioral problems expressed as somatic symptoms or personal distress. From a survey of 118 U.S. medical schools between 1997 and 1999 to which 54 schools responded, topics in biopsychosocial medicine were estimated to constitute approximately 10 percent of medical school curricula (Waldstein et al., 2001).

Additionally, some schools are teaching future physicians about their own mental health needs to prepare them to deal with their feelings about sickness, dying, and death, and several have built self-awareness, personal growth, and well-being activities into their curricula and elective offerings (Novack et al., 1999). At the University of Rochester, for example, the Introduction to Clinical Medicine course, which incorporates parts of the previously taught Biopsychosocial Medicine course, helps students explore how their families and cultures influence their attitudes and motivations by sharing genograms and writing personal illness narratives (Novack et al., 1997). These essential skills and attitudes are further reinforced during the Comprehensive Assessment, a formative evaluation of clinical and basic science knowledge, skills, and attitudes held at the end of the second and third years (Epstein et al., in press). Many such courses are designed to provide students with the skills to monitor their own stress levels and formulate adaptive responses to stress that can help prevent burnout as a student and later as a physician.

In reviewing curricular content across medical schools, it becomes evident that there are great differences in the amount of time spent covering the behavioral and social sciences, that a variety of courses are available, that behavioral and social science content is offered at various times during a student's medical education, and that a wide range of topics is included under the rubric of behavioral and social science (AAMC, 2003a; Milan et al., 1998; Muller, 1984; Waldstein et al., 2001). Additionally, whether or not the behavioral and social sciences are fully integrated into the 4-year program depends on the institution. In 2000, 8 percent of the 62 U.S. medical schools that responded to a survey about their curricula reported having integrated programs of behavioral medicine that stressed the effects of human behavior on health and illness using a biopsychosocial model (Brook et al., 2000). The University of California, San Francisco, is one school that uses an integrated curriculum incorporating the behavioral and social sciences and culture with basic biological and clinical training (Carpenter, 2001; Satterfield et al., 2004). Similarly, the Doctoring course at the University of California, Los Angeles, integrates behavioral and social science material by addressing topics at the intersection of medicine, the patient, and society (Wilkes et al., 1998).

Just as medical schools offer a wide range of content in the behavioral and social sciences, they also use a variety of teaching methods to impart that content. Currently, no national survey or database compiles this information. However, data on teaching methods are available for some specific topic areas, such as communication, and these data indicate that small-group discussions and seminars are the methods most commonly used to teach basic communication skills (see Table 2-1). For psychosomatic medicine, among the vast majority of the 54 medical schools that responded to the above-mentioned curriculum survey, most courses appear to follow a lecture or seminar format (Waldstein et al., 2001).

BARRIERS TO SYSTEMATIC ANALYSIS OF THE BEHAVIORAL AND SOCIAL SCIENCES IN MEDICAL SCHOOL CURRICULA

A broad range of courses in the behavioral and social sciences have been incorporated into medical school curricula as a result of increasing concern that a focus on the biomedical aspects of disease may erode physicians' humanistic attitudes; awareness of social, cultural, and environmental determinants of health; and ability to discriminate between technically possible and morally permissible

TABLE 2-1 Methods for Teaching Basic Communication Skills

Teaching Methods in Use	Percentage of 89 Schools Reporting[*]
Small-group discussions/seminars	91
Lectures/presentations	82
Student interviews with simulated patients	79
Student observations of faculty with real patients	74
Student interviews with real patients	72
Role-playing with peers	60
Rounds	45
Video trigger tapes for discussion	43
Videotapes of student interactions	40
Instructional videotapes	30
Required attendance at community activities	24
Journals (i.e., written reflections)	19
Patient advocacy	14
Storytelling by students	14
Storytelling by patients (i.e., patient narrative)	10

[*]Of the 110 North American medical schools that reported teaching basic communication skills at some point within their curricula, 89 completed the second-stage survey section on teaching methods. The percentages in this table are based on responses from those 89 institutions. Teaching methods are listed if at least 5 percent of the respondents in this sample reported using them.
SOURCE: Adapted from AAMC (1999b).

interventions (Benbassat et al., 2003). Given this diversity, it is difficult to ascertain the precise behavioral and social science content offered and the approaches used to incorporate that content into the curriculum.

One reason the data are difficult to analyze is that the behavioral and social sciences comprise a variety of disciplines, each with its own technology, language, and concepts (Bolman, 1995). How the behavioral and social sciences are defined and which of their aspects have been described in published reports will determine which courses are included in the analysis. For the purposes of this report, the behavioral and social sciences as applied to medicine are ideally defined as those research-based disciplines that provide physicians with empirically verifiable knowledge that serves as a foundation for understanding and influencing individual, group, and societal actions relevant to improving and maintaining health.

Another challenge that arises in reporting what medical schools are teaching students is that some behavioral and social science learning is incidental to the primary information being taught, cannot easily be identified and entered into a database, and is difficult to document and categorize. This is the case even though such incidental learning can profoundly influence a medical student's knowledge, skills, and attitudes. For example, medical students' views of depression may be influenced more by their observation of how a supervising physician handles patients with depressive symptoms than by anything they hear in a lecture or read in a textbook. The teaching that occurs in this format is sometimes referred to as the "hidden curriculum," which can be described as the implicit message continually being conveyed to students through a supervisor's or a role model's example, rather than the person's spoken words. It also involves the imprinting of attitudes and values onto impressionable students by their more-experienced educators (Ludmerer, 1999).

The lack of standardized course content and teaching methods in the behavioral and social sciences leads to the variability among medical schools noted above, which is a further impediment to data collection and analysis. The Liaison Committee on Medical Education (LCME), the accrediting body for U.S. and Canadian medical schools, tracks a number of special topics of relevance to the behavioral and social science content of medical school curricula. However, as is true for other special topic areas, it does not specify how the behavioral and social sciences should be taught, the number of hours a school should devote to these disciplines, or what topics should be covered. It merely states that the curriculum must include behavioral and socioeconomic subjects in addition to basic science and clinical disciplines (LCME, 2003). As a result, each medical school has great flexibility in designing an appropriate program for itself. The lack of a standard program design, however, hampers the systematic analysis of curricular content across medical schools, and makes it impossible to ensure that the most essential and empirically supported behavioral and social science content is included in medical school curricula.

Use of the national database for medical school curricula of the Association of American Medical Colleges (AAMC) does not resolve these difficulties. AAMC's Curriculum Management and Information Tool (CurrMIT) database is the most comprehensive tool available for collecting and analyzing the content of medical school curricula. It is a voluntary system designed to allow medical schools to examine the full spectrum of their course offerings, track key trends, support new innovations, and compare local curricula with those of other medical schools (AAMC, 2003b). Schools have flexibility in the way they enter their data, depending on program needs. As a result, data entry formats vary from school to school, as do the degree to which the information is updated and the level of detail entered (e.g., only 67 schools have provided course titles).

The CurrMIT database lists 142 accredited medical schools (126 in the United States and 16 in Canada). Of these 142 schools, 55 have entered data reporting that the school offers a course in behavioral or social science (AAMC, personal communication, June 2003).

Because LCME requires medical school curricula to include behavioral and socioeconomic subjects (LCME, 2003), it can be assumed that all accredited medical schools in the United States teach behavioral and social science topics in some form. The CurrMIT database may not identify all schools with behavioral and social science courses because not all schools provided the information (AAMC, 2003a) or because the course content and teaching methods could not be identified from the course title. Dartmouth Medical School, for example, offers a course during the second year called On Doctoring that aims to improve students' communication skills through participating in small-group role-playing, visiting patients, and using standardized patients[2] (Cochran and Schiffman, 2003; Dube et al., 2000). However, a search of course titles for the word "communication" would yield a list on which Dartmouth would not appear, whereas the University of Pittsburgh School of Medicine would be included because it offers a course entitled Cell Communication and Signaling (AAMC, 2003a).

This example demonstrates the impossibility of using currently available data to conduct a systematic review of behavioral and social science content in the curricula of the 126 U.S. medical schools. To compound these difficulties, unless medical school data are regularly updated in the only current national database (CurrMIT), they cannot be considered accurate or useful for analyzing the state of behavioral and social science education in medical schools. A change in funding, for example, can drastically alter course content, faculty, and teaching methods, even though the curriculum and course titles may remain the same. In fact, a study at the University of Kansas found a 30–37 percent discrepancy between what course directors say is being taught about prevention in the curriculum and what trained student observers have witnessed in the class (Dismuke and McClary, 2000).

INVENTORY OF CURRENT BEHAVIORAL AND SOCIAL SCIENCE CONTENT IN MEDICAL SCHOOL CURRICULA

Within the limitations of the available data, as described above, the committee pursued its charge of taking an inventory of current behavioral and social science content in medical school curricula by compiling the available data and using indicators to signify the presence, intensity, location, and adequacy of such content. Tables 2-2a, b, and c summarize the results of these efforts. Although it would be desirable to compare the data in these three tables, such analysis is not recommended given that the data come from different sources that utilize varying collection methods and data analyses.

The "Selected LCME Hot Topics" column in each table lists some of the topics on which the LCME focuses in the medical school self-study that is conducted the year before a formal accreditation visit and at the accreditation visit itself. The committee chose these topics as the framework for examining the state of the behavioral and social sciences in medical school curricula because they are

---

[2]Individuals who portray patients with specific medical conditions so students can be trained and evaluated in their ability to interact with patients.

TABLE 2-2a Number of Hours Selected LCME Hot Topics Are Taught Throughout the 4 Years of Medical School

Selected LCME Hot Topics	Mean No. of Hours Taught ± Standard Deviation (no. of schools providing data)
Communication Skills	46±45 (105)
Community Health	28±40 (94)
Cultural Diversity*	15±24 (100)
End-of-Life Care	20±22 (102)
Palliative Care*	12±15 (96)
Epidemiology*	16±11 (110)
Health Care Quality Improvement	4±4 (74)
Health Care Systems*	10±9 (99)
Human Development/ Life Cycle	23±21 (106)
Medical Ethics*	25±19 (109)
Medical Socioeconomics	6±9 (85)
Nutrition	20±15 (106)
Pain Management	10±16 (103)
Palliative Care*	12±15 (96)
Patient Health Education	10±16 (95)
Population-Based Medicine	1±19 (98)
Prevention and Health Maintenance*	22±26 (103)
Substance Abuse	14±15 (106)

*These data are published in Barzansky and Etzel (2003).
SOURCE: LCME 2002-2003 Annual Medical School Questionnaire.

the only subject matter–related content domains with which one can query the LCME national data, the CurrMIT database, and the data from an AAMC-administered survey of graduating students' satisfaction with their educational experiences by subject matter (the Graduation Questionnaire, administered annually to all graduating medical students).

The committee identified the topics that have a prima facie relationship to behavioral and social science content; these appear in bold in the tables. Although many of these topics do not necessarily denote behavioral and social science subject matter, the committee assumed that if they were taught in a contemporary medical school, they would likely involve teaching or at least making reference to information from the behavioral and social sciences. Nutrition is one such example, as the major challenges of obesity and eating disorders involve managing behavioral change and cannot be taught effectively without including content in the behavioral and social sciences. Likewise, because clinical epidemiology is focused on medical decision making and the structuring of information to enable evidence-based clinical inferences and choices, that subject cannot be taught ap-

TABLE 2-2b Percentage of Medical Schools Teaching Specific Topics During Each Year of Medical School

Selected LCME Hot Topics[a]	Percentage[b]			
	Year 1	Year 2	Year 3	Year 4
Communication Skills	51	27	15	3
Patient interviewing skills	39	27	6	2
Doctor–patient communication skills	2	3	3	0
Community Health	15	12	8	5
Cultural Diversity	13	0	0	0
Cultural competency	15	5	2	2
End-of-Life Care	60	52	13	16
Palliative Care	–	–	–	–
Epidemiology	40	49	8	12
Clinical epidemiology	9	9	0	0
Health Care Quality Improvement	5	2	2	2
Health Care Systems	15	8	2	3
Human Development/ Life Cycle	31	16	2	2
Medical Ethics	70	51	22	13
Biomedical ethics	3	0	2	0
Medical Socioeconomics	–	–	–	–
Medical economics	12	13	3	3
Nutrition	75	75	28	8
Pain Management	–	–	–	–
Combined Pain and Palliative Care	72	78	36	19
Patient Health Education	8	6	2	2
Population-Based Medicine	11	15	5	2
Prevention and Health Maintenance	39	45	13	5
Substance Abuse	–	–	–	–
Drug and alcohol abuse	49	81	24	12

NOTE: Data based on 67 medical schools that entered over 200 session titles in the CurrMIT database. "–" indicates data not available.

[a]LCME Hot Topics are shown in bold. Subheadings under those topics represent the closest match to the Hot Topic and Medical School Graduation Questionnaire variables (see Table that can be found in the AAMC CurrMit database).

[b]Percentages calculated from the total number of schools teaching the topic/total number of schools.
SOURCE: AAMC CurrMIT database.

propriately without addressing the psychology and cognitive structure of clinical decision making (Fletcher et al., 1998).

Table 2-2a shows the mean number of hours devoted to teaching each topic and the number of schools on which this mean is based. This mean value is an indicator of the "intensity" of teaching in each behavioral and social science area for which data are available. It should be noted that hours taught may be reported for each topic without the available hours attributable to each having been parsed. For example, if a portion of the clinical communication course were dedicated to

TABLE 2-2c Medical Student Satisfaction with Selected Topics at Time of Graduation

Selected LCME Hot Topics	Percentage N = 14,200
Percentage of students who believe the time devoted to instruction in this area was appropriate	
Communication Skills	
Patient interviewing skills/doctor–patient communication skills	89/88
End-of-Life Care	68
Palliative Care	67
Health Care Quality Improvement	
Quality assurance in medicine	55
Nutrition	36
Pain Management	45
Percentage of students who believe the time devoted to instruction in the area was appropriate	
Population-Based Medicine	
Population-based role of community health and social service agencies	61
Substance Abuse	
Drug and alcohol abuse	86
Percentage of students who believe the subject was adequately covered in all 4 years of medical school	
Community Health	56
Cultural Diversity	
Cultural competency	59
Epidemiology	
Clinical epidemiology	58
Health Care Systems	30
Medical Ethics	
Biomedical ethics	70
Medical Socioeconomics	
Medical economics	17
Prevention and Health Maintenance	
Health promotion and disease prevention	68

NOTE: LCME Hot Topics are shown in bold. Subheadings under those topics represent the closest match to the LCME Hot Topic as it appears on the Medical School Graduation Questionnaire.
SOURCE: 2002–2003 AAMC Graduation Questionnaire (AAMC, 2003c).

discussion of informed consent, this time would be reported under both "communication skills on challenging issues" and "ethical decision making." A grand total of hours is therefore not reported.

Table 2-2b presents indicator measures of the year of medical school in which the various topics are taught. There are several major limitations to interpreting these data. First, as noted earlier, the reporting of curricular content to the CurrMIT database is voluntary, and the data used by AAMC staff to determine the indicator measures are from only 67 of the 126 U.S. medical schools. Next, even within the universe of schools that do report data to the CurrMIT database, more information about the curriculum is generally made available for years 1 and 2 (the preclinical years) than for years 3 and 4 (the clinical years). Therefore, the lower prevalence of teaching specifically focused on hot topics related to the behavioral and social sciences in the third and fourth years is particularly vulnerable to inaccuracy, especially to being underestimated. The best use of the data on the percentage of medical schools teaching specific topics, then, is to compare the prevalence of teaching activity from one topic area to another (up and down the column). It should be noted that some teaching of the topics listed does occur across all 4 years, at least in some schools.

Finally, data in Table 2-2c are from the AAMC Graduation Questionnaire. Nearly all students complete this questionnaire because many schools use the data for educational quality improvement efforts and make completion of the survey a prerequisite for graduation.

After reviewing the data in these tables, the committee made the following observations. First, the data in Table 2-2a reveal substantial variations in the behavioral and social science topics taught in medical school curricula. In the topic domains for which LCME data were available, the topics with the greatest representation (inclusion in the curricula) appear to be communication skills, epidemiology, human development/life cycle, medical ethics, substance abuse, and nutrition. Among these topics, clinical communication skills are reported as receiving the most curriculum time—nearly twice as much as any other topic. The topics that appear to have the least representation and number of required hours within the curricula are health care quality improvement and medical (socio)economics. Even in schools reporting that these topics have a place in the curriculum, the total number of required hours on these topics is small.

The committee also observed that although the data in Table 2-2b are based on only 67 medical schools, it appears that most of the teaching across all the topics listed takes place in the first 2 years of the undergraduate medical curriculum, with some topics (e.g., epidemiology, prevention, and substance abuse) being better represented in the second year than in the first. Other topics (e.g., communication skills, human development/life cycle, and medical ethics) show the reverse pattern. Although the data indicating the extension of these topics into the third and fourth years are incomplete, it is noteworthy that some of the topics (e.g., communication, palliative care/pain management, nutrition, medical ethics, and substance abuse) do demonstrate a proclivity for integration into clinical clerkships. In addition, it would be desirable to know the correlation between overall student satisfaction with specific topics listed in Table 2-2c and other variables, such as the number of hours those topics are taught (Table 2-2a) and the frequency with which the topics are reinforced throughout the 4 years of medical education (Table 2-2b).

APPROACHES OF SELECTED MEDICAL SCHOOLS TO INTEGRATING BEHAVIORAL AND SOCIAL SCIENCE CONTENT INTO THEIR CURRICULA

To supplement information on curricular content and pedagogic methods available in the published literature, the committee conducted brief, ad hoc surveys of four selected medical schools. (For a more-detailed discussion of the methods used to obtain data on behavioral and social science content in medical school curricula, see Appendix A.) The four schools were the University of California, San Francisco, School of Medicine; University of Rochester School of Medicine; Ohio State University College of Medicine and Public Health; and University of North Carolina School of Medicine.

The survey was designed to obtain more in-depth information on the behavioral and social science content in medical school curricula today and to gather further information on useful approaches being taken by medical schools to incorporate such content. Given the constantly changing nature of medical school courses and curricula, the committee believed it important to communicate directly with a sampling of schools to obtain detailed information on their most recent experience with enhancing behavioral and social science content in their curricula. The contacted schools did not constitute a random sample, but became known to the committee in the course of its work as schools with different and substantial achievements in the incorporation of behavioral and social science topics into their curricula. The committee was, however, particularly impressed with the behavioral and social science curricula at the University of Rochester and the University of California, San Francisco. Box 2-1 lists schools with such programs as identified in the literature and through websites. Although this is not an exhaustive list, it does provide a small inventory of schools that can be contacted for more detail on the present state of their instruction in the behavioral and social sciences.

The above four schools were asked to complete a brief written questionnaire and identify a knowledgeable individual at their institution from whom supplemental information could be elicited in a telephone interview. (For a copy of the questionnaire, see Appendix A.) The resulting information is presented in Boxes 2-2 through 2-5. The charts following each box detail the behavioral and social science education provided at each of the schools. It should be noted that the information presented is strictly descriptive and not intended to be representative;

BOX 2-1
Schools with Educational Programs in the
Behavioral and Social Sciences,
Based on the Literature and Website Information

Brown University, School of Medicine (Dube et al., 2000)
Case Western Reserve University School of Medicine (Yedidia et al., 2003)
Dartmouth Medical School (Rabinowitz et al., 2001)
Drexel University, College of Medicine (Drexel University, 2003)
Emory University, School of Medicine (Branch et al., 2001)
Harvard Medical School (Peters et al., 2000)
New York University School of Medicine (Yedidia et al., 2003)
Northwestern University Medical School (Makoul et al., 1998)
Ohio State University College of Medicine (Ohio State University, 2003)
Oregon Health Sciences University School of Medicine (Fields et al., 1998)
University of Arizona (Maizes et al., 2002)
University of California, San Francisco (Satterfield et al., 2004)
University of California, Los Angeles (Wilkes et al., 1998)
University of Chicago, Pritzker School of Medicine (Dickstein, 2001)
University of Connecticut, School of Medicine (Rabinowitz et al., 2001)
University of Kentucky, School of Medicine (Dickstein, 2001)
University of Massachusetts Medical School (Pettus, 2002)
University of Nebraska Medical Center (Steele and Susman, 1998)
University of Rochester, School of Medicine (Novack et al., 1999)

---

rather, it is provided to illustrate the diversity of approaches used to integrate the behavioral and social sciences into the curricula of medical schools today.

From the survey responses, it appears that content from the behavioral and social sciences is not entering medical school curricula in the form of dedicated new courses. Instead, it is integrated into existing courses as thematic content. It is sometimes conveyed in lecture form, but often is discussed in facilitated small groups that evaluate cases prepared for problem-based learning exercises. For advocates of the inclusion of social and behavioral science content in medical school curricula, an encouraging fact is that it does not appear difficult to find course vehicles for lectures or problem-based learning exercises on such topics. Faculty respondents did cite difficulty, however, in determining what social and behavioral science information should serve as core content for lectures or case studies.

BOX 2-2
Behavioral and Social Science Education in the
Medical School Curriculum of Ohio State University

At the Ohio State University College of Medicine and Public Health, teaching of the behavioral and social sciences occurs primarily in a few concentrated courses, with some integration between courses and with other components of the curriculum (see table that follows). Integration occurs, for example, between the courses Patient-Centered Medicine and Senior Partners, and between the teaching of addiction through lectures and small groups and learning in the neural sciences in the basic science curriculum.

Most behavioral and social science issues are presented to students in the Patient-Centered Medicine course, which is offered during the first 2 years. The course is taught once a week through a blend of 1.5-hour large-group lectures and 1.5-hour small-group, case-based sessions. A core group of primary care physicians (mainly from the Family Medicine Department) serve as the small-group facilitators who lead discussions on cases written by a team of educators. The facilitators work with the same group of students over the entire academic year and use teaching modules that include professionalism, palliative medicine, and professional well-being.

Although there is minimal faculty development for facilitators in the behavioral and social sciences, there is some formal education on how to conduct small-group discussions. The director of the Patient-Centered Medicine course observes teachers in small-group sessions and provides feedback.

Ohio State University, College of Medicine and Public Health

Topic	Course(s)	Responsible Department(s)	Year(s) Taught	Teaching Method*
Communication skills	• Doctor–Patient Relationship • Advanced Clinical Interviewing	• Course Director: Family Medicine • Taught by multiple clinical departments	1, 2	SG
Community health	• Patient-Centered Medicine • Working with senior partners • Integrated pathway	• Family Medicine • Geriatrics • Allied Medicine	1, 2, 3, 4	L, O—community project and senior partners
Cultural diversity	• Patient-Centered Medicine	• Family Medicine	1	SG, L

Ohio State University, College of Medicine and Public Health

Topic	Course(s)	Responsible Department(s)	Year(s) Taught	Teaching Method*
End-of-life care	• Patient-Centered Medicine • Working with senior partners	• Anesthesiology • Family Medicine • Geriatrics	1, 2, 3, 4	SG, L, O—senior partners
Epidemiology	• Integrated pathway	• Allied Medicine	1	SG, L
Family/domestic violence	• Patient-Centered Medicine • Clerkships	• Pediatrics • Family Medicine • Obstetrics/ Gynecology	1, 3	SG, L
Health care quality improvement	• Integrated pathway	• General Internal Medicine	2	L
Health care systems	• Integrated pathway	• Allied Medicine	2	L
Health literacy	• Patient-Centered Medicine	• Family Medicine	1	L
Human development/ life cycle	• Patient-Centered Medicine • Pediatric clerkship	• Pediatrics • Family Medicine		SG, L
Medical social economics	• Integrated pathway	• General Internal Medicine	2	L
Pain management	• Patient-Centered Medicine • Integrated pathway	• Anesthesiology • Neurology • Family Medicine	1, 2	SG, L
Palliative care	• Patient-Centered Medicine • Working with senior partners	• Anesthesiology • Family Medicine • Geriatrics	1, 2, 3, 4	SG, L, O—senior partners
Patient health education	• Multiple clerkships	• Anesthesiology • Family Medicine • Geriatrics	3, 4	O—clerkships
Population-based medicine	• Integrated pathway	• Allied Medicine	1	L
Prevention and health maintenance	• Integrated pathway	• Multiple Clerkships	1, 3, 4,	L, O—clerkships
Substance abuse	• Patient-Centered Medicine • Integrative pathway • Ambulatory clerkship • 4th year elective	• Family Medicine • Neurology • Internal Medicine	1, 2, 3, 4	SG, L, O—elective

*L = lecture, PBL = problem-based learning, SG = small group, U = unknown, O = other (describe).

BOX 2-3
Behavioral and Social Science Education in the Medical School Curriculum of the University of California, San Francisco (UCSF)

A dramatically new undergraduate medical curriculum was launched at UCSF in September 2001 (see table that follows). The traditional structure of 2 years of basic sciences plus 2 years of clinical rotations was replaced by a model divided into three stages spanning 4 years: the Essential Core, the Clinical Core, and Advanced Studies. The basic science classes taught during the first 2 years were replaced by courses taught over 16 months of integrated blocks, each centered on clinical cases. Cases taken from primary, secondary, and tertiary care not only illustrate clinical manifestations of disease, but also provide an integrative vehicle for the basic, social, and behavioral sciences. The second phase of the curriculum, the Clinical Core, encompasses 44 weeks of clinical clerkships interspersed with 4 weeks of intersessions, an important innovation that provides critical time for reflection, integration, and consolidation. The third phase, Advanced Studies (34 weeks), gives students a wide selection of elective choices. These include the opportunity to return to basic science, more time for independent scholarly and creative pursuits, the opportunity to gain teaching skills, and opportunities for subspecialty rotations.

An overarching goal of the new curriculum is to practice evidence-based teaching using educational literature that describes how medical knowledge and skills can best be learned, retained, and applied. Essential Core didactic lectures normally do not exceed 2 hours per day, and are usually followed by 2 hours of small-group or laboratory work. Students are encouraged to be active learners through the use of problem-based learning; integrated learning modules (electronic self-guided study materials); and the use of a fully interactive, web-based curriculum.

"The interaction of biology and the environment in determining health" was established as the foundational theme for the new curriculum, opening the way for the meaningful inclusion of behavioral and social science content. A special behavioral and social sciences working group identified five broad sociocultural themes and three behavioral themes to span all nine Essential Core blocks, with the intent to eventually extend these themes into the clerkships and advanced-study years. Sociocultural themes include (1) patterns of health and disease across populations; (2) ethnicity, gender, age, socioeconomic status, and health; (3) the cultures of medicine and health care institutions; (4) physician–patient relationships; and (5) the experience of illness and/or health. The three behavioral themes are (1) stress, distress, and coping; (2) understanding and facilitating behavior change; and (3) personality and social context. Each theme starts with basic attitudes and knowledge as informed by block objectives and active clinical cases, but quickly moves to complex, clinical applications. Demonstration of clinical significance and relevance to medical practice are provided by sharing epidemiologic data, case studies, and master clinician testimonials.

Primary teaching methods used for behavioral and social science content include didactic lectures, typically tied to active learning cases; "teachable moments" integrated into basic or clinical science lectures; multidisciplinary discussion panels; master clinician wrap-ups; guided small-group exercises; and special student projects. Full block calendars, session outlines, learning objectives, and samples of teaching materials can be found at http://medschool.ucsf.edu/ilios/.

The quality of the behavioral and social sciences curriculum was evaluated by examining student performance and conducting student "town hall" meetings, focus groups, and electronic student evaluations. A behavioral and social sciences student advisory board gathered feedback on behavioral and social science classes and provided suggestions for future improvements. Student performance on behavioral and social science content was evaluated through standard multiple-choice questions; short-answer questions; essay exams; and special applied projects, such as dietary self-monitoring, preparation of a biopsychosocial discharge plan; role-plays for smoking cessation; and dietary counseling for a diabetic patient. In the near future, a competency-based, comprehensive assessment for behavioral and social science and other objectives will be implemented at the end of year 2 using adapted Observed Structured Clinical Exams (OSCEs) and standardized patients. Assessment data will be used to revise and improve the existing behavioral and social science curriculum and to extend all behavioral and social science themes into the Clinical Core and beyond.

University of California, San Francisco, School of Medicine

Topic	Course(s)	Responsible Department(s)	Year(s) Taught	Teaching Method*
Communication skills	• Foundations of Patient Care • Multiple clerkships	• Family and Community Medicine • Psychiatry • Medicine • Anthropology, History, and Social Medicine	1, 2, 3, 4	SG, L
Community health	• Foundations of Patient Care • Family and community medicine clerkship	• Family and Community Medicine • Psychiatry • Anthropology, History, and Social Medicine	1, 2, 3	SG, L
Cultural diversity	• Foundations of Patient Care • Block courses: Prologue, Organs, Cancer, Metabolism and Nutrition, Life Cycle	• Family and Community Medicine • Psychiatry • Medicine • Anthropology, History, and Social Medicine	1, 2	PBL, SG, L
End-of-life care	• Foundations of Patient Care • Block courses: Cancer, Life Cycle • Multiple clerkships	• Family and Community Medicine • Psychiatry • Medicine • Anthropology, History, and Social Medicine	1, 2, 3, 4	PBL, SG, L
Epidemiology	• Block courses: Organs, Cancer, Life Cycle, Integration and Consolidation	• Epidemiology	1, 2	SG, L
Family/domestic violence	• Foundations of Patient Care • Block courses: Brain, Mind, and Behavior; Life Cycle	• Family and Community Medicine • Psychiatry • Medicine • Anthropology, History, and Social Medicine	1, 2	SG, L

University of California, San Francisco, School of Medicine

Topic	Course(s)	Responsible Department(s)	Year(s) Taught	Teaching Method*
Health care quality improvement	• Foundations of Patient Care • Block courses: Brain, Mind, and Behavior; Life Cycle	• Family and Community Medicine • Psychiatry • Pediatrics • Anthropology, History, and Social Medicine	1, 2	SG, L
Health care systems	• Foundations of Patient Care • Block courses: Infection, Immunity and Inflammation; Metabolism and Nutrition • Clinical core intersessions	• Family and Community Medicine • Medicine, • Anthropology, History, and Social Medicine	1, 2, 3	PBL, SG, L
Health literacy	• Block course: Prologue	• Anthropology, History, and Social Medicine	1	SG, L
Human development/ life cycle	• Foundations of Patient Care • Block courses: Organs; Life Cycle • Multiple clerkships	• Family and Community Medicine • Psychiatry • Pediatrics • Medicine • Anthropology, History, and Social Medicine	1, 2, 3, 4	PBL, SG, L
Medical social economics	• Foundations of Patient Care • Block course: Prologue	• Family and Community Medicine • Anthropology, History, and Social Medicine	1, 2	SG, L
Pain management	• Block courses: Organs; Life Cycle • Multiple clerkships	• Family and Community Medicine • Pediatrics • Medicine	1, 2, 3, 4	SG, L

Continued

University of California, San Francisco, School of Medicine

Topic	Course(s)	Responsible Department(s)	Year(s) Taught	Teaching Method*
Palliative care	• Block courses: Cancer, Life Cycle • Multiple clerkships	• Family and Community Medicine • Psychiatry • Pediatrics • Medicine	1, 2, 3, 4	SG, L
Patient health education	• Foundations of Patient care • Multiple clerkships	• Family and Community Medicine • Psychiatry • Pediatrics • Medicine • Anthropology, History, and Social Medicine	1, 2, 3, 4	SG, L
Population-based medicine	• Block courses: Prologue; Organs; Cancer; Brain, Mind and Behavior; Infection, Immunity, and Inflammation	• Family and Community Medicine • Epidemiology • Medicine • Anthropology, History, and Social Medicine		
Prevention and health maintenance	• Foundations of Patient Care • Block courses: Prologue; Organs; Cancer; Infection, Immunity, and Inflammation; Metabolism and Nutrition; Life Cycle; Integration and Consolidation • Multiple clerkships	• Family and Community Medicine • Psychiatry • Pediatrics • Medicine • Anthropology, History, and Social Medicine	1, 2, 3, 4	SG, L
Substance abuse	• Block courses: Brain, Mind, and Behavior; Infection, Immunity, and Inflammation; Life Cycle	• Family and Community Medicine • Psychiatry • Pediatrics • Medicine • Anthropology, History, and Social Medicine	1, 2	SG, L

*L = lecture, PBL = problem-based learning, SG = small group, U = unknown, O = other (describe).

BOX 2-4
Behavioral and Social Science Education in the
Medical School Curriculum of the University of Rochester

The Double Helix Curriculum (DHC) at the University of Rochester School of Medicine and Dentistry was built on the strong tradition of biopsychosocial medicine that has been a hallmark of a Rochester education since the 1940s (see table that follows). The goal is to produce patient-centered physicians who maintain a passion for lifelong learning and are able to keep pace with the biomedical advances that influence the study and clinical practice of medicine.

With this goal in mind, the DHC weaves basic science and clinical strands across all 4 years of undergraduate medical education. Pharmacology, pathology, and genetics, for example, do not exist as separate courses but are incorporated in every course in the curriculum. In recognition of the essential role of the behavioral and social sciences in the practice of medicine, six themes are integrated throughout the curriculum. These themes (aging, diversity, ethics and law, health economics, nutrition, and prevention) are often "orphan topics" at many schools. At Rochester, however, each of these themes has specific learning objectives for each course and year. Many of the core behavioral and social science topics are addressed within the learning objectives for these themes. Faculty theme directors work with course and clerkship directors in the development of problem-based learning cases, as well as in the creation of innovative learning opportunities for behavioral and social science topics.

Additional core behavioral and social science topics are covered in other courses and clerkships throughout the DHC. The initial medical school course at Rochester is entitled Mastering Medical Information. In this course, students not only learn about medical informatics, epidemiology, and biostatistics, but also begin to study aspects of nutrition and diversity through problem-based learning cases. The first component of the Ambulatory Clerkship emphasizes prevention and health maintenance. In addition to building on their interviewing and physical examination skills, students learn and practice behavioral medicine skills, such as smoking cessation counseling, alcohol and drug screening and counseling, diet and exercise counseling, and adolescent health maintenance topics, in primary care offices.

Behavioral and social science topics in year 2 are emphasized in the context of the integrated neuroscience course, entitled Mind, Brain and Behavior, and in the integrated pathophysiology course, entitled Disease Processes and Therapeutics. Near the end of year 2, students participate in a formative comprehensive assessment, which emphasizes basic

continued

BOX 2-4 Continued

science topics in a clinical setting utilizing a variety of assessment methods, including standardized patients, computer-based exams, and a team-based evaluation with an anesthesia simulator. The comprehensive assessment pays significant attention to students' communication and counseling skills, which have been honed over the course of the Ambulatory Clerkship. Additionally, it examines the student's ability to integrate essential behavioral and social science topics encompassed by courses, clerkships, and themes.

Behavioral and social science coursework is also incorporated in years 3 and 4 of the DHC through clerkship directors' attention to the theme learning objectives. Moreover, another formative comprehensive assessment is completed at the end of year 3, in which students are able to assess their growth and development over the year. The DHC also includes a required year 4 Community Health Improvement Clerkship that is tied to the community health mission of the University of Rochester Medical Center. This clerkship provides students with an opportunity not only to engage in structured service learning, but also to learn more about related health economics, health disparities, and diversity, essential topics in today's health care environment.

Rochester's long-standing tradition in biopsychosocial medicine and patient-centered care has a renewed emphasis in the DHC. The outcomes of the relatively new curriculum are being followed through regular internal evaluation of themes, courses, and clerkships, as well as review of external assessments, including the AAMC Graduation Questionnaire results and student performance on the U.S. Medical Licensing Examination.

University of Rochester, School of Medicine

Topic	Course(s)	Responsible Department(s)	Year(s) Taught	Teaching Method*
Communication skills	• Introduction to Clinical Medicine • Ambulatory clerkship	• Internal Medicine • Family Medicine • Psychiatry	1, 2	SG, L
Community health	• Mastering Medical Information • Ambulatory clerkship—community health • Improvement clerkship	• Community and Preventive Medicine • Internal Medicine • Family Medicine • Psychiatry	1, 2, 4	PBL, SG, L

University of Rochester, School of Medicine

Topic	Course(s)	Responsible Department(s)	Year(s) Taught	Teaching Method*
Cultural diversity	• Diversity theme • Addressed in problem-based learning cases within courses in years 1 and 2	• Multiple departments	1, 2, 3, 4	PBL, SG, L
End-of-life care	• Ambulatory clerkship • Ethics and law theme • Aging theme	• Internal Medicine • Family Medicine • Pediatrics • Medical Humanities	2, 3	SG, L
Epidemiology	• Mastering Medical Information	• Community and Preventive Medicine	1	PBL, L
Family/domestic violence	• Ambulatory clerkship • Emergency medicine clerkship	• Internal Medicine • Family Medicine • Emergency Medicine • Pediatrics	2, 4	L, O
Health care quality improvement	• Health economics theme • Year 2 case seminars • Successful Interning	• Neurology • Community and Preventive • Internal Medicine	2	PBL, L
Health care systems	• Health economics theme • Year 2 case seminars	• Neurology • Community and Preventive Medicine • Internal Medicine	2	PBL, L
Health literacy	—	—	—	—
Human development/ life cycle	• Introduction to Clinical Medicine • Mind, Brain and Behavior • Ambulatory clerkship	• Internal Medicine • Family Medicine • Pediatrics • Psychiatry	1, 2, 3	PBL, L
Medical social economics	—	—	—	—

Continued

University of Rochester, School of Medicine

Topic	Course(s)	Responsible Department(s)	Year(s) Taught	Teaching Method*
Pain management	• Ambulatory clerkship • Inpatient clerkships	• Internal Medicine • Family Medicine • Pediatrics • Pharmacology/ Physiology	2, 3	PBL, SG, L
Palliative care	• Ambulatory clerkship • Ethics and law theme • Inpatient clerkships • Electives	• Internal Medicine • Family Medicine • Pediatrics • Medical Humanities • Nursing	2, 3	SG, L
Patient health education	—	—	—	—
Population-based medicine	• Mastering Medical Information • Community health improvement clerkship	• Community and Preventive Medicine	1, 4	PBL, L, O
Prevention and health maintenance	• Ambulatory clerkship • Mastering Medical Information • Nutrition theme	• Internal Medicine • Family Medicine • Pediatrics • Community and Preventive Medicine	1	SG, L
Substance abuse	• Ambulatory clerkship • Mind, Brain and Behavior • Psychiatry clerkship	• Internal Medicine • Family Medicine • Pediatrics • Neurology • Psychiatry	1, 2, 3	PBL, SG, L

*L = lecture, PBL = problem-based learning, SG = small group, U = unknown, O = other (describe).

BOX 2-5
Behavioral and Social Science Education in the
Medical School Curriculum of the
University of North Carolina

The Department of Social Medicine is the primary source of behavioral and social science education for medical students at the University of North Carolina School of Medicine. Behavioral and social science material is integrated as a content theme across several courses in the curriculum and is taught as a content theme in six required courses: two in year 1 and four in year 2 (see table that follows).

In the Medicine and Society course, offered through the Department of Social Medicine in year 1, there are no examinations, but students are required to participate in creative writing assignments and engage in group discussions that teach a habit of critical reflection using the tools of the social sciences and humanities. Cultural diversity, end-of-life care, and medical social economics are some examples of the behavioral and social science topics discussed in the course. Selection of small-group leaders for the Medicine and Society course is fairly competitive and requires a strong commitment from faculty as both active learners and teachers. Despite the requirements, many members of the faculty are willing to make the necessary commitments to teach this course. An interdepartmental course that complements Medicine and Society—Introduction to Clinical Medicine—is directed by the dean's office. The faculties that teach both courses are careful to distinguish between the courses: Medicine and Society is not trying to teach specific skills, and Introduction to Clinical Medicine is not attempting to teach social science theory or concepts; rather, the two courses run in parallel and draw from each other. This sort of coordination is facilitated by the dean's office, which brings course directors together on a monthly basis.

University of North Carolina, School of Medicine, Social Medicine Department

Topic	Course(s)	Responsible Department(s)	Year(s) Taught	Teaching Method*
Communication skills	• Introduction to Clinical Medicine 1 (ICM-1) • ICM-2 • Clinical Epidemiology • Various clerkships	• Dean's Office (ICM) • Social Medicine • Medicine, Pediatrics, Family Medicine, Obstetrics/ Gynecology clerkships	1, 2, 3	PBL, SG, O— one-on-one on medical wards
Community health	• ICM-1 and ICM-2 • Medicine and Society (M&S) • M&S (1st year) • Family Medicine, Pediatrics, and Obstetrics/ Gynecology clerkships • Ambulatory care selective (4th year)	• Dean's Office (ICM) • Social Medicine • Family Medicine • Pediatrics • Obstetrics/ Gynecology	1, 2, 3, 4	PBL, SG, O— experience in communities
Cultural diversity	• ICM-1 and ICM-2 • M&S • Various clerkships	• (Dean's Office) ICM • Social Medicine • Various clinical departments	1, 2, 3	SG
End-of-life care	• M&S • Special Topics day (1st year) • Humanities and Social Science (HSS) Seminar selective • Medicine, Family Medicine, and Obstetrics/ Gynecology clerkships	• Social Medicine • Dean's Office • Social Medicine • Internal Medicine • Family Medicine • Obstetrics/ Gynecology	1, 2, 3	SG, L
Epidemiology	• Clinical Epidemiology • Medicine clerkship	• Social Medicine • Internal Medicine	2, 3	PBL, SG

University of North Carolina, School of Medicine, Social Medicine Department

Topic	Course(s)	Responsible Department(s)	Year(s) Taught	Teaching Method*
Family/domestic violence	• Special Topics day (1st year) • Clinical Epidemiology • Family Medicine, Pediatrics, and Obstetrics/ Gynecology clerkships	• Dean's Office • Social Medicine • Family Medicine • Pediatrics • Obstetrics/ Gynecology	1, 2, 3	PBL, SG, L
Health care quality improvement	• M&S (1st year) • HSS selective	• Social Medicine	1	PBL, SG
Health care systems	• M&S (1st year) • HSS selective	• Social Medicine	1	PBL, SG
Health literacy	• ICM-1 and ICM-2 • Clinical Epidemiology • Medicine Clerkship	• Dean's Office • Social Medicine • Internal Medicine	1, 2, 3	SG
Human development/ life cycle	• Family Medicine, Pediatrics, and Obstetrics/ Gynecology, and Internal Medicine clerkships	• Family Medicine • Pediatrics • Obstetrics/ Gynecology • Internal Medicine	3	
Medical social economics	• M&S (1st year) • HSS selective	• Social Medicine	1	PBL, SG, L
Pain management	• Surgery, Obstetrics/ Gynecology, and Internal Medicine	• Surgery • Obstetrics/ Gynecology • Internal Medicine	3	—
Palliative care	• Internal Medicine • Family Medicine, Obstetrics/ Gynecology, and Surgery clerkships	• Internal Medicine • Family Medicine • Obstetrics/ Gynecology • Surgery	3	
Patient health education	• ICM-1 and ICM-2 • Pediatrics, Obstetrics/ Gynecology, and Family Medicine	• Dean's Office • Pediatrics • Obstetrics/ Gynecology • Family Medicine	1, 2, 3	PBL, SG

Continued

University of North Carolina, School of Medicine, Social Medicine Department

Topic	Course(s)	Responsible Department(s)	Year(s) Taught	Teaching Method*
Population-based medicine	• Some students (5–10/year) take a year off between the 3rd and 4th years of medical school and complete a master's of public health in the School of Public Health. Many also do community service projects.			
Prevention and health maintenance	• ICM-1 and ICM-2 • Clinical Epidemiology • Family Medicine, Pediatrics, Medicine, and Obstetrics/ Gynecology	• Dean's Office • Social Medicine • Family Medicine • Pediatrics • Internal Medicine • Obstetrics/ Gynecology	1, 2, 3	PBL, SG, L
Substance abuse	• Special Topics day (1st year) • Family Medicine, Medicine, Obstetrics/ Gynecology, and Pediatrics clerkships	• Dean's Office • Family Medicine • Medicine • Obstetrics/ Gynecology • Pediatrics	1, 3	PBL, SG, L
Determinants of health (extra-credit question)	• M&S	• Social Medicine	1	SG, L
Human sexuality (extra-credit question)	• Special Topics day (1st year) • HSS selective* • Reproductive Medicine	• Dean's Office • Social Medicine • Obstetrics/ Gynecology	1, 2	PBL, SG, L

*L = lecture, PBL = problem-based learning, SG = small group, U = unknown, O = other (describe).

A recognizable challenge is also apparent in the area of faculty development. Because the facilitators of problem-based learning exercises are typically generalist faculty or specialists who are not themselves behavioral or social scientists, they require training in behavioral and social science content before they can effectively facilitate student learning in these small-group discussions. Individuals from three of the four schools surveyed—University of California, San Francisco; University of Rochester; and Ohio State University—acknowledged a need for more faculty development. The fourth school, University of North Carolina, has a 26-year history of well-supported curriculum innovation in the behavioral and social sciences and a faculty that possesses the needed expertise. That expertise is the product of many years of experience in providing faculty training, coteaching arrangements that pair generalists with behavioral and social science specialists, and regular updates in the behavioral and social sciences for faculty who participate in this curriculum. A particularly noteworthy finding from interviews of individuals from the three other schools was that formal faculty development in the behavioral and social sciences does not generally occur, often because of constraints on faculty time.

At these exemplar schools, the overall faculty response to new behavioral and social science content in the curriculum has generally been favorable. The strongest advocates of this content are the faculty participants in the courses that serve as vehicles for the new content. The interviews also revealed a somewhat less-favorable attitude toward such content by basic science faculty whose preclinical courses are often being downsized not because of the new behavioral and social science content per se, but because the objectives of overall curriculum reform often include providing students with more time for self-directed learning. The attitude toward new behavioral and social science content among students has generally been favorable. There are some examples of new courses that have become extraordinarily popular with students, partly because of the introduction of new behavioral and social science content and partly because of the use of innovative teaching methods.

Overall, the results of these surveys and interviews reveal both similarities and some distinctive differences in the behavioral and social science content in the four institutions' curricula. The general dynamics and challenges of their curriculum and faculty development can be seen at all schools (and are dealt with more extensively in Chapter 4 of this report). The distinctive approaches taken to incorporate the behavioral and social sciences, on the other hand, are representative of the enduring missions and traditions of these schools, which establish the framework within which change is encouraged and accommodated.

NEED FOR AN IMPROVED DATABASE ON THE STATUS OF BEHAVIORAL AND SOCIAL SCIENCE INSTRUCTION IN U.S. MEDICAL SCHOOLS

The review of the current literature and the available data conducted for this report revealed that medical school courses incorporating the behavioral and social sciences vary greatly in their titles, the teaching methods used, and the hours devoted to these topics. This variation reflects the breadth of the behavioral and social sciences and their application to the practice of medicine, the differing needs of communities, and the preferences and expertise of faculty members. National empirical data based on voluntary reporting by schools of medicine (from the CurrMIT database) and accreditation data (from LCME) confirm the variability in subject matter from topic to topic and school to school. The lack of national standardization among medical school curricula, of standardization in the terminology used to describe curricular content, and of a comprehensive strategy for creating a national database of medical school curricula makes it difficult to describe systematically the subject matter medical schools have incorporated into their curricula.

The committee believes the creation of an improved, periodically updated database for information on the state of behavioral and social science instruction in U.S. medical schools would be of significant benefit. An alternative to creating a new database would be to modify CurrMIT to produce these data. Because both are major undertakings, the decision to develop a new database or modify CurrMIT should be based on which method best collects behavioral and social science teaching information within the available resources. Individual medical schools could use this database to compare their coverage of the behavioral and social sciences with that of other institutions to determine whether their curricular content, teaching methods, or means of evaluating student performance need revision. Credentialing bodies could use the database to compare what is actually being taught with the subject matter that is assessed by their evaluation instruments. Government agencies and professional organizations concerned with improving the quality of behavioral and social science instruction and ensuring that new physicians have been exposed to important research findings would also find the database helpful.

The committee believes AAMC is the logical organization to design and operate such a database, as it has access to and is respected by all U.S. allopathic medical schools, and its staff has considerable experience and expertise in data collection and analysis. AAMC should consider collaborating with other relevant professional organizations, such as the American Association of Colleges of Osteopathic Medicine and LCME, in the design and operation of the database.

It is beyond the scope of the committee's charge to specify the data that should be collected, the collection methodology, or the types of analyses that should be performed—matters that would best be decided by those using the database. It may be noted that the ad hoc survey conducted by the committee for this study reflects some of its thinking about the minimum contents of a curriculum database.

Conclusion 1. *Existing national databases provide inadequate information on behavioral and social science content, teaching techniques, and assessment methodologies. This lack of data impedes the ability to reach conclusions about the current state and adequacy of behavioral and social science instruction in U.S. medical schools.*

Recommendation 1: *Develop and maintain a database.* **The National Institutes of Health's Office of Behavioral and Social Sciences Research should contract with the Association of American Medical Colleges to develop and maintain a database on behavioral and social science curricular content, teaching techniques, and assessment methodologies in U.S. medical schools. This database should be updated on a regular basis.**

3

The Behavioral and Social Sciences in Medical School Curricula

TASK 2: *Develop a list of prioritized topics from the behavioral and social sciences for possible inclusion in medical school curricula. As an alternative to a numerical list, clustered priorities (e.g., top, high, medium, low) may be assigned to topic areas.*

SUMMARY: *Adverse health effects can be created or exacerbated by harmful behaviors (smoking, poor diet, sedentary lifestyle, excessive alcohol consumption, and risky sexual behaviors). Similarly, psychological, social, biological, and behavioral factors have been shown to influence disease risk and illness recurrence. Such mind–body interactions and behavioral influences on health and disease are important concepts to which medical students should be exposed. Students should also graduate with an understanding of how their background and beliefs can affect patient care and their own well-being; how they can best interact with patients and their families; how cultural issues influence health care; and how social factors, such as health policy and economics, affect physicians' ability to provide optimal care for their patients.*

Practicing physicians need to be skilled in all 26 of the priority topics identified in this chapter. Because medical education is a continuum, it is neither necessary nor desirable for medical students to become experts in every priority topic. By graduation, however, students should be able to demonstrate competency in the six domains described in this report and at a minimum have an understanding of the 20 high-priority topics within those domains. These topics should be reinforced throughout the 4 years of medical school. To what depth the 26 priority topics are taught and evaluated will vary according to the focus and needs of the particular medical school.

No physician's education would be complete without an understanding of the role played by behavioral and social factors in human health and disease, knowledge of the ways in which these factors can be modified, and an appreciation of how personal life experiences influence physician–patient relationships. The committee believes that each medical school should expect entering students to have completed course work in the behavioral and social sciences during their prebaccalaureate education and should inform prospective applicants of its behavioral and social science–related requirements and/or recommendations. Behavioral and social science instruction in medical school should build on this prebaccalaureate foundation. The committee also believes that material from the behavioral and social sciences should be included in the post–medical school phases of the medical education continuum. These phases include residency and fellowship training, as well as continuing (postgraduate) medical education. While the emphasis in this report is on the 4 years of medical school, the importance of continuing behavioral and social science education throughout a physician's career cannot be overemphasized.

This chapter responds to the second part of the committee's charge—to develop a list of prioritized topics from the behavioral and social sciences for possible inclusion in medical school curricula. The committee considers this to be the most important part of its work. Before presenting the prioritized topics, however, the committee offers two conclusions reached during its deliberations.

Conclusion 2a. *Human health and illness are influenced by multiple interacting biological, psychological, social, cultural, behavioral, and economic factors. The behavioral and social sciences have contributed a great deal of research-based knowledge in each of these areas that can inform physicians' approaches to prevention, diagnosis, and patient care.*

Some areas of the behavioral and social sciences have been more thoroughly researched and rigorously tested than others. This observation does not diminish the importance of those areas with less verifiable evidence, but rather points to the need for more research. One such example is the strong influence physicians' actions can have on the attitudes and values of medical students, even though this nonverbal form of communication has not been thoroughly tested (Ludmerer, 1999). In contrast, the importance of effective physician communication has received a fair amount of attention by researchers. The results of this research indicate that physicians need basic communication skills in order to take accurate patient histories, build therapeutic relationships, and engage patients in an educative process of shared decision making (IOM, 2001a, 2003a; Peterson et al., 1992; Safran et al., 1998).

Conclusion 2b. *Within the clinical encounter, certain interactional competencies are critically related to the effectiveness and subsequent outcomes of health care. These competencies include the taking of the medical history, communication, counseling, and behavioral management.*

Before attempting to identify the specific topics in the behavioral and social sciences to which medical students should be exposed, the committee considered ways in which material from these disciplines might be included in the curriculum. Experiences at the medical schools of the University of California, San Francisco, at the University of Pennsylvania, and at the University of Rochester, among others (UCSF, 2003; University of Rochester, 2002), have shown that an effective way to present the behavioral and social sciences to medical students is in an integrated manner throughout the 4 years of medical school, rather than confining this material to the preclinical years. Providing this content over the 4 years of medical school will introduce it at a time when students perceive it to be most relevant and facilitate reinforcement of important concepts throughout the preclinical and clinical years. Moreover, integrating the curriculum so that behavioral and social science topics are included as part of other basic science and clinical courses, instead of being presented in separate courses, will enable the educational experience to simulate real-world experience, in which behavioral and social factors in health and disease must be considered in the context of complex clinical situations.

In formulating recommendations for core content in the behavioral and social sciences, the committee was aware that the current medical school curriculum is extremely full. The committee therefore attempted to limit its recommendations to those items it believes are most important and should be covered at a relatively early stage in a physician's education. The presentation of additional material, as well as reinforcement of the material covered in medical school, could be reserved for later stages of the medical education continuum. The committee also recognized that it had neither the license nor the time to delineate a detailed curriculum (specific methods of instruction, detailed content, and the appropriate time to introduce various items) in the behavioral and social sciences. Formulation of a curriculum is the responsibility of medical school faculties, and the recommendations made in this report might be incorporated into a curriculum in a number of different ways. Innovation and the diversity it produces have been strengths of the American medical education system, and should apply to the behavioral and social sciences as well as to other components of the medical school curriculum.

To formulate the priorities recommended in this report, the committee developed an extensive list of possible behavioral and social science topics on the basis of a number of sources and considerations:

int evidence-based articles and reports in the literature

ations to the committee by content experts and medical school rep-

ure and other materials from the Association of American Medical
\MC) and the Liaison Committee on Medical Education

∟∪∩siderations related to the health of the public, driven mainly by root
causes of morbidity and mortality

- The gap between what is known and what is actually done in practice

Following extensive deliberations, the committee used a modified Delphi
process to prioritize this initial list. (A detailed description of this process is included in Appendix A.) Committee members rated each of the topics on the list
using a scale system, and then assigned each high, medium, or low priority based
on its mean score and standard deviation. This list was further refined and finalized using the collective and individual experience of the committee as experts in
medical school curriculum development and reform in the behavioral and social
sciences. The low priorities were then discarded, and the remaining 26 topics
were categorized as top, high, or medium priority. The results of this process
constitute the committee's recommendation for those behavioral and social science topics that should be included in medical school curricula. In the committee's
view, the 20 topics ranked top and high must be included in medical school curricula and were therefore combined into one high-priority group. The 6 medium-
priority topics are also important and would significantly enhance the education
of medical students. Inclusion of the medium priorities, as well as the depth of
teaching and evaluation, is dependent upon the needs of the individual medical
school.

The final listing of topics, presented in Table 3-1, is organized so as to have
meaning for medical school curriculum committees. The 26 recommended topics
fall into the following 6 general domains of knowledge:[1]

- *Mind–body interactions in health and disease*—focuses on the four primary pathways of disease (biological, behavioral, psychological, and social). Students need to recognize and understand the many complex interactions among
these pathways that may be compromising a patient's physical and/or mental
health.
- *Patient behavior*—centers on behavioral pathways to promoting health
and preventing disease. Educating medical students about behaviors that pose a
risk to health will better equip them to provide appropriate interventions and
influence patient behavior.

---

[1]The order in which the various domains are listed is random, and does not reflect the committee's
view of their relative importance.

TABLE 3-1 Behavioral and Social Science Topics of High and Medium Priority for Inclusion in Medical School Curricula

Domain	High Priority	Medium Priority
Mind–Body Interactions in Health and Disease	• Biological mediators between psychological and social factors and health • Psychological, social, and behavioral factors in chronic disease • Psychological and social aspects of human development that influence disease and illness • Psychosocial aspects of pain	• Psychosocial, biological, and management issues in somatization • Interaction among illness, family dynamics, and culture
Patient Behavior	• Health risk behaviors • Principles of behavior change • Impact of psychosocial stressors and psychiatric disorders on manifestations of other illnesses and on health behavior	
Physician Role and Behavior	• Ethical guidelines for professional behavior • Personal values, attitudes, and biases as they influence patient care • Physician well-being • Social accountability and responsibility • Work in health care teams and organizations • Use of and linkage with community resources to enhance patient care	
Physician–Patient Interactions	• Basic communication skills • Complex communication skills	• Context of patient's social and economic situation, capacity for self-care, and ability to participate in shared decision making • Management of difficult or problematic physician–patient interactions
Social and Cultural Issues in Health Care	• Impact of social inequalities in health care and the social factors that are determinants of health outcomes • Cultural competency	• Role of complementary and alternative medicine
Health Policy and Economics	• Overview of U.S. health care system • Economic incentives affecting patients' health-related behaviors • Costs, cost-effectiveness, and physician responses to financial incentives	• Variations in care

- *Physician role and behavior*—emphasizes the physician's personal background and beliefs as they may affect patient care, as well as the physician's own well-being.
- *Physician–patient interactions*—focuses on the ability to communicate effectively, which, as noted above, is a critical component of the practice of medicine.
- *Social and cultural issues in health care*—addresses what physicians need to know and do to provide appropriate care to patients with differing social, cultural, and economic backgrounds.
- *Health policy and economics*—includes those topics to which medical students should be exposed to help them understand the health care system in which they will eventually practice (although additional material regarding the U.S. health care system should be presented in the residency years).

Recommendation 2. *Provide an integrated 4-year curriculum in the behavioral and social sciences.* **Medical students should be provided with an integrated curriculum in the behavioral and social sciences throughout the 4 years of medical school. At a minimum, this curriculum should include the high-priority items delineated in this report and summarized in Table 3-1. Medical students should demonstrate competency in the following domains:**

- **Mind–body interactions in health and disease**
- **Patient behavior**
- **Physician role and behavior**
- **Physician–patient interactions**
- **Social and cultural issues in health care**
- **Health policy and economics**

MIND–BODY INTERACTIONS IN HEALTH AND DISEASE

High Priority

- Biological mediators between psychological and social factors and health
- Psychological, social, and behavioral factors in chronic disease
- Psychological and social aspects of human development that influence disease and illness
- Psychosocial aspects of pain

Medium Priority

- Psychosocial, biological, and management issues in somatization
- Interaction among illness, family dynamics, and culture

High-Priority Topics

Biological Mediators Between Psychological and Social Factors and Health

Research in psychosomatic medicine has documented how disease and illness are related to many potentially interacting causes. These can include biological insults (e.g., carcinogens and microbes), genetic susceptibility, early childhood experiences, personality, acute and chronic stressors, behaviors, socioeconomic status, and lifestyle. Comprehensive reviews of this science have recently been published by committees of the National Research Council and the Institute of Medicine (IOM, 2001b; NRC, 2001). A large body of research has established the presence of biological mediators between such factors and health. These include genetic mediators, as well as those of the central nervous system, the autonomic nervous system, and the endocrine and immune systems (IOM, 2001b; McEwen, 2002; NRC, 2001).

To achieve a more comprehensive understanding of the maintenance of health and the genesis of disease, therefore, students need to learn the basics of psychophysiology, that is, how stressors and a variety of psychological, behavioral, and social factors alter physiology to make disease more likely, and how the systems that maintain homeostasis are interconnected and can react to various stressors in concert. For example, psychoneuroimmunology is the study of the interconnections among the central nervous system, the neuroendocrine system, and the immune system and the implications of those connections for the ways in which stress, emotions, and psychology affect immune function. Acute stress tends to enhance that function by promoting immune cell translocation to sites of immune challenge, whereas chronic stress (through the mediation of hormonal factors) tends to have a deleterious effect on immune function and disease processes

(Dhabhar and McEwen, 1999). The relationship between stress and the immune system has been demonstrated in animal models, which have shown that stress makes animals more vulnerable to experimental tumors (Ben-Eliyahu et al., 1991) and infections (Ben-Nathan and Feuerstein, 1990; Ben-Nathan et al., 1991; Bonneau et al., 1991; Friedman et al., 1965; Rasmussen et al., 1957).

Research with humans also has shown that immune function may be altered by affective states and by major and minor acute and chronic stressful life experiences (Biondi, 2001). Chronic stress and a lack of social support, for example, increase the likelihood that a person will develop a cold after being challenged with a standard dose of a rhinovirus (Cohen, 1995). In addition, stress-induced modulation of the immune system has been linked to the expression of inflammatory, infectious, and autoimmune diseases.

Psychological, Social, and Behavioral Factors in Chronic Disease

In the year 2000, roughly 125 million Americans—nearly half of the U.S. population—were living with some type of chronic condition (Partnership for Solutions, 2003). Sedentary lifestyles, poor dietary habits, and the large population of aging baby boomers have all contributed to the rising rates of age- and lifestyle-related chronic medical conditions, such as diabetes, heart disease, and arthritis. The number of cancer patients has grown steadily over the past two decades, and these patients are surviving longer than ever before as a result of improvements in early detection and treatment of the disease. Likewise, the widespread use of potent combination antiretroviral therapy has led to a growing population of people living with HIV infection, who retain a potentially lifelong risk of spreading this infection to others (IOM, 2003b).

These trends have led to recognition that medical students must be educated in the psychological, social, and behavioral factors that can potentially lead to chronic medical conditions and in the interplay between these factors and particular chronic illnesses. For example, it is strongly believed that hostility, chronic stress, depression, social isolation, and increased use of alcohol and tobacco are related to an elevated risk of coronary heart disease (Barefoot et al., 2000; Carroll et al., 1976; Frasure-Smith et al., 1993; Kawachi et al., 1996; Orth-Gomer et al., 1993). Conversely, changing behaviors that may place a person at risk of myocardial infarction, such as hostility and impatience, can reduce the risk of reinfarction in post-myocardial infarction patients (Friedman et al., 1986; Mendes de Leon et al., 1991). Studies have also shown that psychological and social factors influence the development and course of cancer (Everson et al., 1996; Watson et al., 1999).

Other behaviors, such as engaging in risky sexual practices or sharing needles with an HIV-infected partner, significantly affect whether an uninfected patient will contract HIV. Medical students should know which individuals are at greatest risk of becoming infected with HIV and which are most likely to continue to engage in risky behaviors after becoming infected, especially if they do not show outward signs of disease. Students should also be educated in how to recognize distress in chronically ill patients. For example, HIV-infected individuals who exhibit signs of persistent depression have been shown to have increased rates of mortality (Ickovics et al., 2001; Mayne et al., 1996), and stressful life events have been shown to cause a faster progression from HIV-positive status to AIDS (Leserman et al., 2000).

Psychological and Social Aspects of Human Development That Influence Disease and Illness

Human development is the product of the elaborate interplay of biological, psychological, and social influences (U.S. DHHS, 1999), and disease and illness can be understood more fully when the combined effects of these factors are considered at different life stages (Hertzman and Power, 2003; Power and Hertzman, 1997). Exposure of the developing brain to severe or prolonged stress, for example, may result in anatomical and biological changes that can have profound effects lasting throughout the individual's life (Charmandari et al., 2003; Weinstock, 1997). Abnormalities may appear in childhood, adolescence, and adulthood as excessive fear and addictive behaviors, dysthymia and/or depression, and symptoms of metabolic X syndrome (Charmandari et al., 2003; Tsigos and Chrousos, 2002).

Life-cycle theories of Sigmund Freud, Jean Piaget, Erik Erikson, John Bowlby, and others on human development through infancy, toddlerhood, middle childhood, adolescence, adulthood, and old age help physicians understand the process of maturation from a variety of perspectives. Medical students should be exposed to these theories, as well as to their basic underlying principle—the Epigenetic Principle of the Lifecycle Theory—which states that the foundation for each step along the path to maturity is laid by the conditions and events that precede it (Kaplan et al., 1994). This is one of the compelling theories and approaches to adult development, and may fit well into the behavioral and social science portion of a medical school curriculum.

Psychosocial Aspects of Pain

Pain is the most common reason that people consult a physician (HBCC, 1993). There has been growing recognition that pain is a complex perceptual experience influenced by a wide range of psychosocial factors that can include emotions; social and environmental conditions; sociocultural background; personal experiences, beliefs, attitudes, and expectations; and biological factors (Turk and Okifuji, 2002). There is evidence that many physicians undertreat pain (Cleeland, 1998; Portenoy and Lesage, 1999). Furthermore, physician biases may play a role in the undertreatment of pain in patients from certain minority ethnic groups (Cleeland et al., 1997; Todd et al., 1993). Medical students need to develop a solid understanding of the concept that pain is a multidimensional experience with sensory, affective, and behavioral components.

Melzack and Wall's (1965) gate-control theory of pain focuses on the basic anatomy and physiology of pain and provides a conceptual basis for understanding how psychological and behavioral processes exert their effects on the pain experience. Recent findings from functional and anatomical studies provide support for a new perspective that views pain as a homeostatic emotion that integrates both specific neural elements and convergent somatic activity (Craig, 2003). When there is an obvious physical cause for pain, such as in cancer or surgical patients, treatment through pharmacotherapy may be indicated. Anxiety, however, may exacerbate pain, and apparent symptoms of pain can develop in the context of emotionally stressful situations, such as job loss, low levels of social support, or marital difficulties (Krantz and Ostergren, 2000). Consequently, behavioral or cognitive techniques can be useful in combination with medication in treating pain in such patients. In the case of patients with chronic pain without a clear somatic abnormality, a functional analysis is useful for determining the factors eliciting the pain (Drossman, 1978; Kroenke and Swindle, 2000).

Medical students should learn that culture is among the factors that can affect patients' expression of pain. For example, certain ethnic groups have a tendency to express and describe physical complaints in a more dramatic manner than other ethnic groups who may be more apt to accept and conceal pain (Galianti, 1997). In either case, there is a risk that a patient's pain may go untreated, depending on how it is expressed and interpreted by the physician. The International Association for the Study of Pain has published a useful outline of a curriculum on pain for medical school education (Pilowsky, 1988).

Medium-Priority Topics

Psychosocial, Biological, and Management Issues in Somatization

Somatization is the tendency to experience, conceptualize, and communicate mental states and distress as physical symptoms or altered bodily function (Singh, 1998) and is commonly observed in medical practice (Bridges and Goldberg, 1985; Kroenke, 1992). The symptoms produced by somatization are among the leading reasons for medical outpatient clinic visits, with the most common symptoms, such as headache and fatigue, having a prevalence of 10 percent or more. Such common symptoms are frequently related to emotional stress. Affective illnesses such as anxiety and depression, which are frequently undiagnosed by primary care physicians, often present with somatic manifestations (Katon, 1984; Katon and Russo, 1989).

Physicians who fail to make organic diagnoses may label their patients as "somatizing," "problem patients," or even "hateful," which results in patients feeling rejected.

No single theory adequately explains somatization (Kellner, 1990). A biopsychosocial approach to the phenomenon could help students understand how a variety of factors can lead to the presentation of somatic distress (Epstein et al., 1999). Students should understand the diagnostic criteria for somatoform disorders, the many somatic manifestations of affective disorders, and how analysis of their own reactions to patients can help them recognize possible somatoform disorders in their patients. They should also understand how to use the physician–patient relationship as a therapeutic tool for these patients (Hahn et al., 1994; Novack, 1987).

Early recognition and appropriate management of somatization may prevent needless medical workups, doctor shopping, and a further decline in health (Singh, 1998). A number of effective therapeutic strategies for somatoform disorders have been outlined (Barsky and Borus, 1999; Drossman, 1978; Goldberg et al., 1992), and students should be familiar with these and other approaches (Epstein et al., 1999).

Interactions Among Illness, Family Dynamics, and Culture

Family dynamics and culture have a significant influence on a person's perception and expression of illness. In many cultures, for example, an HIV or AIDS diagnosis is perceived as shameful (Paxton, 2000). These feelings of shame and guilt can prevent infected patients from disclosing their HIV status to their families, with the result that they experience isolation and depression at a time when family support is most needed (Black and Miles, 2002; Kadushin, 2000; Kalichman et al., 2003). Physicians must be taught that such cultural biases can influence many aspects of medical treatment. In the case of mental illness, cultural factors influence whether a distressed person seeks help, what type of care is sought, what coping styles are employed, and how much stigma the patient attaches to his or her condition (U.S. DHHS, 1999). Culture also influences the meanings people attribute to their illness. Among some African Americans, Alzheimer's disease is believed to reflect a life of worry and strain that affects the mind in old age (Dilworth-Anderson and Gibson, 2002). In Asian families, dementia is often viewed as an internal imbalance or lack of harmony. These interpretations of illness affect the type of medical care sought. Moreover, patient, sibling, and parental ages and the developmental stages of each family member affect when, where, and how care is sought, as well as how patients' symptoms are manifested (Christ, 2000; Henderson and Gutierrez-Mayka, 1992; King and Dixon, 1996; Montgomery et al., 2002; Ritchie, 2001; Rothchild, 1994; Schiffrin, 2001; Sholevar and Perkel, 1990).

Medical students should learn to recognize how families and the communities in which patients live give meaning to illnesses and how this meaning affects their patients' health and treatment decisions. They should also understand the importance of eliciting familial and cultural information that can positively or negatively influence their patients' medical care.

PATIENT BEHAVIOR

High Priority

- Health risk behaviors
- Principles of behavior change
- Impact of psychosocial stressors and psychiatric disorders on manifestations of other illnesses and on health behavior

High-Priority Topics

Health Risk Behaviors

Numerous behaviors influence health. The six behaviors discussed below are included here because they are currently the major causes of morbidity and mortality in the United States, especially among youth (Kann et al., 1996). At a minimum, medical students should be knowledgeable about the psychosocial factors associated with the development and maintenance of these six behaviors that place their patients at risk, and should become skilled in assessing their patients for these behaviors. They should also understand key strategies for the prevention and cessation of behaviors that pose a health risk, and in particular should be aware of the role of the health care provider in instigating and maintaining changes in such behaviors.

Tobacco use. Cigarette smoking is the major cause of preventable morbidity and mortality in the United States. Overall, smoking causes more than 430,000 deaths per year in this country alone (U.S. DHHS, 2000b). It causes coronary heart disease (NHLBI, 2003b; Wilson et al., 1998); chronic obstructive pulmonary disease (NHLBI, 2003a); and cancers of the lung, larynx, esophagus, pharynx, mouth, and bladder (U.S. DHHS, 2000b). It is also the most important modifiable cause of poor pregnancy outcomes in the United States (Hoyert, 1996).

The prevalence of smoking among the U.S. population is currently about 23 percent, although in some population subgroups, such as those with low educational attainment, the prevalence is between 26 and 38 percent (NCHS, 2003a). Effective treatment programs are available for smoking cessation, including both behavioral and pharmacological components. It is recommended that at every health care encounter, health care providers deliver brief counseling on smoking cessation and offer pharmacotherapy and follow-up to all users of tobacco products (Fiore et al., 2000).

Physical inactivity, poor diet, and obesity. The combination of physical inactivity and detrimental dietary patterns, including excess caloric intake, is the second most important factor contributing to mortality and morbidity in the United States (McGinnis and Foege, 1993; Mokdad et al., 2004). Sedentary lifestyles have been linked to 23 percent of deaths from major chronic diseases, while dietary factors are associated with 4 of the 10 leading causes of death—coronary heart disease, stroke, type II diabetes, and some forms of cancer (Hahn et al., 1990). Obesity, which is often linked to physical inactivity and poor diet, is a major factor in type II diabetes (Morsiani et al., 1985). Physical inactivity and obesity are widespread in the United States, where more than 60 percent of adults do not meet current physical activity guidelines, and 61 percent of adults are overweight or obese (U.S. DHHS, 2001).

Excessive alcohol consumption. Long-term excessive use of alcohol increases the risk of hypertension, arrhythmias, cardiomyopathy, and stroke, as well as some cancers (NIAAA, 2002) and poor pregnancy outcomes (Hoyert, 1996). Heavy use of alcohol is a major risk factor for chronic liver disease and cirrhosis (NIAAA, 1998) and is a major contributor to fatalities resulting from motor vehicle accidents. There were 19,358 alcohol-induced deaths in the United States in 2000, not including fatalities from motor vehicle accidents, and 26,552 deaths from chronic liver disease and cirrhosis to which alcohol consumption was a major contributor (Minino et al., 2002; NIAAA, 2002). Yet alcohol use is a complex issue because low levels of alcohol consumption (one drink per day for women, two drinks per day for men) have been shown to have protective health effects for certain diseases (Sacco et al., 1999; Valmadrid et al., 1999). Fully 62 percent of U.S. adults are considered current drinkers at any level of consumption, and 32 percent of current drinkers had five or more drinks on a single occasion at least once in the past year (NCHS, 2002; U.S. DHHS, 2000a).

Risky sexual behavior. Sexually transmitted diseases are especially problematic among adolescents, a group with a high frequency of short-term relationships, and only about 60 percent of adolescents who are currently sexually active regularly use condoms (CDC, 2002b). HIV, the virus that causes AIDS, is transmitted primarily through sexual contact or the sharing of needles among drug users (IOM, 2003b). Efforts to decrease HIV transmission therefore focus on behavioral interventions that minimize high-risk behaviors and decrease exposure to HIV. Other, more common sexually transmitted infections (e.g., human papilloma virus infection, gonorrhea, and chlamydia infection) have also been associated with poor health outcomes, including cancer, infertility, and long-term disability (IOM, 2003b). The Centers for Disease Control and Prevention estimates that in the United States, 700,000 people are infected with chlamydia, and 350,000–400,000 are infected with HIV (CDC, 2003).

Homicides and physical abuse. Homicide is a major cause of death in the United States and is the leading cause of death among Hispanic and non-Hispanic blacks aged 15–24 (CDC, 2002a). Major behavioral and psychosocial factors associated with homicide and domestic violence include poverty, firearm availability, alcohol abuse, drug abuse, and cultural acceptance of violent behavior (Brook et al., 2003). Physical intimidation and violent behavior may occur in the workplace, schools, and the home. Emergency department personnel or patients' personal physicians (e.g., pediatrician or gynecologist) are often the first responsible persons not belonging to the family to become aware that physical abuse is occurring.

Domestic violence is frequently underrecognized in medical practice (Reid and Glasser, 1997). Physicians should regularly inquire about domestic physical abuse because of its high prevalence and high rate of morbidity (Alpert, 1995; Gin et al., 1991; Hamberger et al., 1992; Warshaw, 1997; Warshaw and Alpert, 1999). A history of sexual and physical abuse is common among female patients with functional gastrointestinal disorders and leads to increased rates of health care utilization and medically unexplained symptoms. However, these women rarely disclose this history unless they are asked directly (Leserman and Drossman, 1995; Leserman et al., 1998; Walker et al., 1995). Thus, it is important that physicians be able to ask about such a history comfortably and sensitively when appropriate. Physician education and the simple inclusion of a single question about domestic abuse during the patient interview can significantly improve the rates of recognition of this behavior (Freund et al., 1996; Kripke et al., 1998; Thompson et al., 2000).

Unintentional injuries. Another leading cause of death in the United States is accidents, which peak at ages 15–24 and then rise again after age 60 (NCHS, 2003a). Nearly half of all deaths among young people are related to motor vehicles, whereas falls are the leading cause of unintentional injuries among older people. Young men in particular are prone to unintentional injury, which is often related to high-risk behaviors and alcohol use (Holtzman et al., 2000).

Principles of Behavior Change

Mounting evidence indicates that primary care physicians can be effective in changing patient behavior by using a variety of techniques (Beresford et al., 1997; IOM, 2001b; Nawaz et al., 2000; Wadden et al., 1997; Walker et al., 1981). Often, however, physicians have not received training in such techniques and therefore cannot appreciate how theoretical concepts of behavior change can be operationalized through effective patient counseling. A number of conceptual models (classical conditioning, cognitive social learning theory, health belief model, theory of reasoned action, stages-of-change or transtheoretical model, and social action theory) are available to guide behavior change interventions that address various behavioral attributes (Bandura, 1986; IOM, 2001b; Prochaska and DiClemente, 1986; Williams et al., 1998). Although each of these models has its limitations, they are useful constructs for thinking about behavior change and can be applied to a variety of desirable changes, including adhering to weight loss regimens, actively seeking breast cancer screening, reducing risk-taking sexual activities, and maintaining smoking cessation (Ashing-Giwa, 1999; Farkas et al., 1996; Keller and Allan, 2001).

Learning and conditioning models are among the oldest and most widely researched models. Conditioning models are of particular importance for various aspects of health-related interventions, such as reinforcement, stimulus–response relationships, modeling, cues to action, and expectancies. Medical students should be made aware of the stimulus-control concept, which posits that patients vary their responses according to the situation in which they find themselves. For example, a person may be in the habit of smoking after a meal and may crave cigarettes only after eating lunch or dinner. Likewise, someone who has a drink every day after work grows to expect a drink at that time. By identifying such almost obligatory responses, the physician can target interventions to have a direct impact on the patient's risky behavior.

Positive reinforcement (being rewarded) and negative reinforcement (getting rid of something unpleasant) are also important concepts for medical students to understand. Encompassed by these concepts are avoidance and escape behaviors—actions that make it possible to escape or prevent pain or discomfort. In such cases, a desirable action is reinforced by the relief it provides. Because different patients respond well to different stimuli, it is prudent for physicians to know which reinforcement will most likely produce the desired effect in their patients.

Medical students should have a grasp of the theoretical and empirical foundations of our understanding of how behaviors are acquired, maintained, and eliminated in the context of health risk. They should also possess a basic understanding of how patients' social and economic situations, physical status, and psychological states affect their motivation to change their behavior and how this information can be linked to the appropriate behavior reinforcement method.

Impact of Psychosocial Stressors and Psychiatric Disorders on Manifestations of Other Illnesses and on Health Behavior

In a recent survey, six of seven physicians indicated their belief that people with chronic conditions have unmet mental health needs, and about half said they believe unaddressed emotional problems lead to poorer medical outcomes (Partnership for Solutions, 2003). Psychosocial stressors, such as chronic medical conditions, divorce, and poverty, can lead to psychological disorders, such as anxiety and depression. However, nonpsychiatrists often fail to recognize the co-occurrence of mental distress and physical disorders, even though anxiety and depression usually present with physical symptoms in the general medical setting. About half to two-thirds of patients with multiple (six or more) medically unexplained physical symptoms, such as chest pain, abdominal pain, headache, and back pain, have either an underlying anxiety or depressive disorder (Kroenke, 2003; Kroenke et al., 1994). Such patients are frequently misdiagnosed. One study, for example, found that patients with panic disorder see 10 physicians on average before receiving a correct diagnosis (Sheehan et al., 1980).

To improve their ability to recognize and treat mental disorders and chronic medical illness, medical students must receive education and training in the co-occurrence of the two and the impact of depression and anxiety on the course of comorbid medical conditions. Students need to learn not only the range of effective treatments, but also how to undertake a conversation with their patients about these treatments. They must also know when to initiate treatment as a medical generalist or specialist and when to refer the patient to a psychiatrist.

For example, medical students should learn to screen for depression in patients with chronic disease. The evidence indicates that patients with chronic medical conditions have a high prevalence of major and minor depression (Cassano and Fava, 2002); conversely, older patients with multiple chronic conditions or disabilities experience high rates of depression (Lee et al., 2001). Indeed, evidence suggests that comorbid depression plays a role in the onset and course of several conditions, especially coronary artery disease and congestive heart failure (Januzzi et al., 2000). Likewise, it has been estimated that 10 to 15 percent of patients with diabetes have major depression (Lustman et al., 1998), and it has been found that the severity of depression is associated with the prognosis of the disease (Ciechanowski et al., 2000).

Depression affects a person's ability to function in social and work environments and negatively impacts quality of life and overall well-being. Whooley and Simon (2000) suggest that providers should aggressively treat depressed patients who have other medical problems because depression makes people more vulnerable to somatic distress, results in poorer self-care, and worsens the prognosis for diseases such as cardiovascular disorders. Therefore, it is in the nation's interest to train medical students to understand the pathogenetic relationships between depression and comorbid medical conditions.

PHYSICIAN ROLE AND BEHAVIOR

High Priority

- Ethical guidelines for professional behavior
- Personal values, attitudes, and biases as they influence patient care
- Physician well-being
- Social accountability and responsibility
- Work in health care teams and organizations
- Use of and linkage with community resources to enhance patient care

High-Priority Topics

Ethical Guidelines for Professional Behavior

Violations of professionalism and ethical behavior are the major reasons for physicians losing their licenses (Papadakis et al., 1999). Codes of professional conduct help guide physicians' actions and promote their personal commitment to the welfare of patients, while also informing collective efforts to improve the health care system.

The intent of education in medical ethics is to make explicit and understandable the many ethical and professional dilemmas faced by students and physicians and to offer guidelines on which to base ethical decision making. Many efforts, such as the Medical Professionalism Project sponsored by the American Board of Internal Medicine, have been aimed at identifying fundamental principles of professionalism—including the primacy of patient welfare, patient autonomy, and social justice—and sets of professional responsibilities (ABIM, 2001). A series of commitments to professional competence, honesty, confidentiality, and the establishment of appropriate relations with patients is derived from these principles. Ethical principles are needed in particular to guide practice in the many demanding and often emotionally charged situations and contexts of modern medicine, such as end-of-life treatment and care, withdrawal of life support, and reproductive decision making.

Student experiences in medical school can be used as learning opportunities to teach ethical values. Those experiences might include the need to address such questions as the following:

- When is it acceptable for students to perform procedures on patients to gain experience and skills, although the risk to patients may be greater than it would be if more experienced trainees or graduate physicians were to carry out the same procedures?
- How can students draw the line between acceptable and unacceptable behaviors when senior members of a medical team ask them to engage in actions that misrepresent who accomplished the work (e.g., students completing informed

consents instead of residents or writing progress notes and charts for others), especially in situations in which the students' performance ratings and credentials are at stake?

• How should students challenge inappropriate or even offensive treatment of patients observed in clinical work situations when they are on the lowest rung of the medical decision-making ladder?

• Should students introduce themselves to patients and families as medical students, recognizing that patients may assume that anyone in a white coat is a fully credentialed medical doctor?

These are examples of clinical ethical quandaries that students must resolve, sometimes on their own. All of these value-laden situations demand clear reasoning, an understanding of underlying personal and professional values and basic first principles, well-developed communication skills, and even group leadership skills.

Medical schools have used numerous pedagogical approaches to address such issues. Many of these teaching and learning approaches—such as the use of problem-based cases, small-group exercises, interaction with standardized patients, reading and discussion of materials drawn from the humanities, discussions during clinical rounds, and opportunities to talk with and obtain feedback from senior personnel—are discussed in Chapter 2.

The education for a virtuous life in medicine does not, of course, begin or end in medical school, as many of the scholastic issues faced by medical students (e.g., cheating and plagiarizing) arise earlier. However, medical students first experience the distinct challenges of clinical responsibility in preceptorships and clerkships when they begin to care for patients.

Personal Values, Attitudes, and Biases as They Influence Patient Care

Physicians' attitudes guide their behaviors, and these attitudes are in turn shaped by a variety of factors, including personal histories, family and cultural backgrounds, values, biases, and emotions. Both unrecognized and recognized feelings and attitudes can adversely affect physician–patient communication (Stein, 1985) and may emerge inappropriately during the medical encounter, endangering the physician–patient relationship (Bennett, 1987).

Assuming that physicians develop adequate levels of knowledge and skill through their training, it will be their attitudes that ultimately determine the quality of the care they provide. This includes attitudes about the importance of psychosocial factors in medical care and about the importance of self-sufficiency, personal responsibility, family values, aging, racial and ethnic differences, and death, all of which shape the physician–patient interaction (Carmel, 1997; Cheng et al., 1999; Ely et al., 1998; Epstein et al., 1993; Nightingale et al., 1991; Novack et al., 1997; O'Loughlin et al., 2001).

An individual's family of origin can have a major influence on his or her attitudes (Novack et al., 1997). This is the context in which one first learns about the nature, benefits, and pitfalls of caring; the roles of the caregiver; the balance of giving and receiving; the communication aspects of illness; and how to respond to distress—dynamics that are fundamentally important to the physician–patient relationship. Patients may remind physicians of family members with similar problems or behavioral patterns, eliciting such feelings as fear of harming the patient, being inadequate, or losing control, or discomfort in addressing certain difficult topics (Marshall and Smith, 1995).

Because personal factors can play such an important role in the development of physicians' attitudes, some have stressed the need to emphasize in medical education activities that promote personal awareness (Anonymous, 1969; Epstein, 1999; Lipkin et al., 1995b; Longhurst, 1988; Novack et al., 1997, 1999). It is noted that improved personal awareness facilitates positive relationships with patients (Gorlin and Zucker, 1983; Marshall and Smith, 1995) and the ability to cope with stress (Quill and Williamson, 1990). Physicians who become more aware of the influence of personal factors on their behaviors can better examine how and why they make behavior choices (Stein, 1985). This personal awareness can be a first step in stimulating adaptive changes in attitude and behavior and can also lead to a deeper and more sophisticated understanding of patients' behaviors.

For these reasons, it is essential that medical schools provide opportunities within their curricula for students to reflect upon and discuss how their family of origin, cultural background, gender, life experiences, and other personal factors have influenced their attitudes toward emotional reactions to patients. Students should be offered such structured activities as the Balint method[2] (The Balint Society, 2003; Luban, 1995) and support groups (Brashear, 1987; Williamson, 1992) to help them process the difficult emotional encounters that regularly occur in medical care and to learn from the experiences of peers and teachers.

Physician Well-Being

The stresses of medical training have been well documented. Students are faced with acquiring an overwhelming amount of knowledge in a relatively short period, working long hours, and dealing with occasional abuse on rounds, as well as the suffering and death of patients (Bourgeois et al., 1993; Lubitz and Nguyen,

---

[2]The Balint method consists of regular case discussion in small groups under the guidance of a qualified group leader. The work of the group involves both training and research to help general practitioners gain a better understanding of the emotional content of the doctor–patient relationship. This method has been adapted for use in medical schools.

1996; Silver and Glicken, 1990). Medical education has even been characterized as a "neglectful and abusive family system," promoting cynicism, callousness, and self-doubt (McKegney, 1989:452). A number of the stresses of medical training have been associated with long-term adverse effects on physical health, mental well-being, and work performance measures (Baldwin et al., 1997b; Shanafelt et al., 2002). In addition, many physicians have developed maladaptive responses to stressors and have not appropriately managed their own health care needs (Baldwin et al., 1997a; Martin, 1986).

Studies have documented increased anxiety and depression in large numbers of students upon entering medical school that persists throughout the 4 years (Clark and Zeldow, 1988; Rosal et al., 1997; Vitaliano et al., 1988) and into postgraduate training and physician practice (Clark et al., 1984; Hendrie et al., 1990; Ramirez et al., 1995; Reuben, 1983; Shanafelt et al., 2002; Smith et al., 1986; Vitaliano et al., 1988, 1989). Such high levels of stress often lead to burnout, which has been associated with residents' reports of providing suboptimal patient care and a decreased sense of professional satisfaction (Fields et al., 1995; Shanafelt et al., 2002). Moreover, many trainees and physicians in practice carry work stress home with them, resulting in strained family relationships (Warde et al., 1999); decreased intimacy and greater marital discord (Gabbard and Menninger, 1989); and stress-related somatic complaints, such as headache, backache, fatigue, and atypical chest pain (Geurts et al., 1999).

Medical schools can do much to address the issues of balance and self-care, as well as the prevention of stress, burnout, and impairment in their students. Rigorously designed interventional studies on stress management in medical students have shown that teaching stress reduction techniques can reduce psychological distress and anxiety (Palan and Chandwani, 1989; Shapiro et al., 1998; Whitehouse et al., 1996). These techniques can be used throughout students' medical training and into their medical practice. Students can also be taught to recognize risk factors and warning signs of depression, burnout, substance abuse, and other mental health problems in themselves (Chang et al., 1997; Clark et al., 1984; Firth-Cozens, 2001; Linzer et al., 2001; McCranie and Brandsma, 1988; Shanafelt et al., 2003); to adopt wellness strategies that promote physician well-being (Firth-Cozens, 2001; Quill and Williamson, 1990; Shanafelt et al., 2003; Weiner et al., 2001); to apply principles for creating healthy, intimate relationships (Christie-Seely, 1986; Myers, 2001); to clarify personal values (Clever, 2001); and to openly discuss realistic strategies for creating balance in their lives (Coombs and Virshup, 1994). This can be done both as part of the curriculum and as part of extracurricular activities.

Students learn best when they are physically and emotionally healthy. If they can learn during medical training about attending to balance in their lives and to the prevention, early detection, and treatment of burnout and emotional problems, they can acquire habits that will enhance their lives and their medical practices over the long term.

Social Accountability and Responsibility

A socially responsible individual has been defined as "a person who takes part in activities that contribute to the happiness, health, and prosperity of a community and its members" (Faulkner and McCurdy, 2000:347). Some educators have expressed concern that medical training is not adequately preparing physicians to be socially responsible members of society and that medical schools are not fulfilling their social responsibility to improve the health of the public (Coulehan et al., 2003; Schroeder et al., 1989). AAMC also recognizes that medical schools have a special duty to teach their medical students how to become socially responsible physicians (McCurdy et al., 1997). It is vitally important for educators to understand and nurture the social contract that exists between medical schools and the public.

Defining the elements of a socially accountable and responsible curriculum is difficult and not within the scope of this report, but the committee notes that two fundamental principles should be paramount in medical school curricula. First, medical students should be engaged in activities that foster their development as socially responsible leaders. These activities must extend beyond the doctor–patient relationship to encompass the complex web of multidisciplinary relationships within society. The World Federation for Medical Education has recommended that schools enlarge the range of settings in which educational programs are conducted to include all health resources of the community, not hospitals alone (Anonymous, 1988; Byrne and Wasylenki, 1996). Progress is being made toward accomplishing this goal. Although much of medical education is still conducted in tertiary-care hospitals, medical students are increasingly being exposed to community-based health settings and to organizations that serve the community.

In addition, students must be taught to recognize the priority health concerns of the community, region, and/or nation they serve (Boelen, 1995). Graduates should understand that health care needs change over time and that they must be prepared to respond to the changing needs of the community in which they practice. By continually profiling the health status and health care needs of the community, medical schools can create an awareness in students of the current and emerging needs of their individual communities within the larger context of national and international trends (Parboosingh, 2003). This understanding of community needs can then be reinforced by experiential learning that acquaints students with real-world problems as they engage in socially responsible public service.

Work in Health Care Teams and Organizations

Increasingly, health care is delivered by multidisciplinary teams of professionals that can include physicians, social workers, nurses, nutritionists, and physical and mental health therapists. Each discipline brings a unique perspective to the care of the patient, and physicians must recognize what each has to offer. They must also accept the fact that most health care organizations and institutions no longer embrace the top-down model of medical treatment whereby the physician is the sole decision maker in the patient's care. A doctor who does not interact well with those in other disciplines will likely experience greater difficulty in expediting his or her wishes. It is therefore crucial that physicians know how to work effectively in the context of integrated teams. They must understand their role as part of a team and why it is important to foster positive relationships with other team members.

The chronic care model developed by Wagner and colleagues is an example of how physicians can work effectively in the context of integrated systems and teams (Glasgow et al., 2000, 2001a; Von Korff et al., 1997; Wagner et al., 1996, 2001). Recently, this model has been applied to preventive care as well (Glasgow et al., 2001a,b). The overall goal of the chronic care model is to create an environment that supports productive interactions between informed, activated patients and a prepared, proactive team of clinicians (Von Korff et al., 1997; Wagner et al., 1996, 2001). Exposing medical students to such theoretical models is helpful but not sufficient; medical students should also participate in educational experiences with other health professionals. This type of learning environment fosters communication across health care disciplines and exposes medical students to perspectives other than medicine in the care of patients. Such interdisciplinary learning prepares students for the realities of working in integrated health care teams and organizations and should be reinforced throughout the 4 years of medical school.

Use of and Linkage with Community Resources to Enhance Patient Care

An emphasis on disease prevention and the economic constraints of medical practice and care delivery are often at odds, limiting the time available for providers to devote to preventive care issues. However, a number of community resources can assist health care providers in their efforts to offer preventive services to their patients. These resources may include social work, mental health counseling, and nutrition education services.

Learning about available community resources can help medical students identify valuable health and social services in the patient's community. For example, exposing medical students to a local hospice organization during discussion of end-of-life care provides a natural link to a valuable resource for both patient care and physician information. Numerous community-based programs for behavior counseling and disease prevention and health promotion—such as drug abuse programs, protective services for domestic violence, HIV prevention programs, smoking cessation programs, and nutritional counseling—may be available as well. In addition, some local, state, and federal programs provide access to screening and medical treatment for those with or at risk of developing specific illnesses. Examples include local initiatives for breast and prostate cancer screening for underserved populations (Boyd et al., 2001; Frelix et al., 1999; McCoy et al., 1994). These services provide an opportunity for health care providers to extend their own preventive care efforts and provide access to prevention services for low-income and/or underinsured patients.

Physicians should be aware of the availability of these services in their community and have a working knowledge of the types of interventions offered. While this information can be found through local chapters of voluntary health organizations, social service agencies, and websites of national associations and organizations, students should be made aware during their training of the utility of such allied services in fostering the health of their patients. Remaining current with available community resources is an important element of continuing education.

PHYSICIAN–PATIENT INTERACTIONS

High Priority

- Basic communication skills
- Complex communication skills

Medium Priority

- Context of patient's social and economic situation, capacity for self-care, and ability to participate in shared decision making
- Management of difficult or problematic physician–patient interactions

High-Priority Topics

Basic Communication Skills

Good communication skills are necessary if physicians are to take accurate patient histories, build therapeutic relationships, engage patients in an educative process of shared decision making, and encourage patient adherence to treatment. In fact, 75 to 95 percent of the information needed for physicians to make a correct diagnosis comes from the patient-reported medical history (Gruppen et al., 1988; Peterson et al., 1992), and competent history taking is known to be essential to providing effective care (Matthews et al., 1993; Novack, 1987; Safran et al., 1998; Stewart et al., 1999). The quality and quantity of diagnostic information gathered in the medical interview depend on the physician's approach to interviewing and his or her interviewing skills (Beckman and Frankel, 1984; Marvel et al., 1999).

Conceptual advances and research findings that have emerged in recent decades have radically changed physicians' understanding of the process and teaching of medical interviewing. For example, clinical reasoning can be taught and integrated into medical students' interviewing skills to facilitate successful history taking (Kahn et al., 1979; Makoul, 1998; Novack et al., 1993; Schmidt et al., 1990; Stoeckle and Billings, 1987). These skills include establishing rapport and building trust, eliciting adequate information to permit a robust differential diagnosis, understanding and addressing patient concerns, and initiating patient education and counseling. Medical students who learn these skills have the ability to conduct thorough interviews in a time-efficient manner (Cole and Bird, 2000). A variety of models have been developed to guide students in learning these skills (Cole and Bird, 2000; Coulehan and Block, 2001; Haidet and Paterniti, 2003; Kurtz et al., 1998; Lazare et al., 1995; Lipkin et al., 1995a; Makoul, 1998; Platt and Platt, 2003; Platt et al., 2001; Smith, 1996; Stewart et al., 1995).

Medical students need to acquire skills that promote communication with patients beyond simply asking about their disease symptoms. As emphasized earlier, cultural sensitivity and physician self-awareness are key components of effective communication in this regard (Epstein, 1999; Kleinman et al., 1978; Novack et al., 1997). In addition to the many biomedical questions that must be asked in every standard medical interview, students need to be trained to inquire comfortably about patients' concerns, emotions, social situations, and behaviors (Goldberg and Novack, 1992). Medical students who learn how to elicit information needed to understand how biological, personal, and social factors interact in the onset and maintenance of illness will diagnose and treat their future patients more effectively. In addition, medical students need to understand how to engender a therapeutic relationship and be trained to recognize potential barriers between physician and patient that could endanger this relationship and hinder patient compliance (Lazare et al., 1995; Quill, 1989). Skills needed to accomplish this include expressing empathy (Spiro, 1993); actively listening (Beckman et al., 1994); and eliciting information about patients' lives, as well as their expectations and concerns about their medical care (Levinson et al., 2000; Rao et al., 2000).

Effective communication, together with skilled health behavior counseling, promotes patient adherence to treatment and facilitates changes in patients' problematic or risky health behaviors, including smoking, substance use, and unsafe sexual practices (DiMatteo, 1994a,b; Glasgow et al., 2002; Goldstein et al., 1998; Grueninger et al., 1995; Roter and Kinmonth, 2002; Whitlock et al., 2002). Motivational interviewing (Miller and Rollnick, 2002) is an approach to patient health behavior counseling that integrates principles of patient-centered counseling with established models of health behavior change, including the transtheoretical model, self-determination theory, and social cognitive theory. The technique has been modified for use in clinical settings and is a promising approach to treating problem behaviors (Burke et al., 2003). Students should be exposed to this interviewing technique, as well as the 5As counseling approach (Assess, Advise,

Agree, Assist, Arrange follow-up), which has been recommended by the U.S. Preventive Services Task Force's Counseling and Behavioral Interventions Work Group as a unifying conceptual framework for delivering and evaluating health behavioral counseling interventions in primary and general health care settings (Goldstein et al., 1994; Whitlock et al., 2002).

Complex Communication Skills

Although the basic communication skills needed by physicians for taking an accurate medical history are necessary for every physician–patient encounter, a number of situations require expertise in more-specific areas. A panel of senior faculty of the American Academy on Physician and Patient created a list of clinical encounters that require such specialized knowledge and skills (see Box 3-1) (Novack, 1998). Relevant conceptual and practical issues can be identified for all of these encounters, as can specific strategies and behaviors that will promote effective communication. Because the first two groups (I and II) of items listed in Box 3-1 represent core clinical encounters in medical care, all students upon graduation should be able to demonstrate proficiency in dealing with these encounters. Medical students can learn the basic issues involved in the items listed in groups III and IV, but they would not be expected to attain proficiency in these encounters until residency.

Medium-Priority Topics

Context of a Patient's Social and Economic Situation, Capacity for Self-Care, and Ability to Participate in Shared Decision Making

The personal, social, and economic resources available to patients can affect their ability to participate in shared decision making about their health care. Medical students need to be taught to be aware of their patients' ability to participate in decision making, and, when possible, determine whether the necessary *resources* are available to ensure access to care and avoid obstacles that could impede diagnosis and treatment of a disease.

Personal resources are considered attributes of the individual, and can include age, health status, level of motivation, and education. Social resources encompass primary and secondary relationships that provide sources of social support to patients. Patients who are embedded within strong social support networks (e.g., families and places of religion) often report less depressive symptoms than those who are not (Goldberg et al., 1985). Economic resources, such as employment or income, are those that enable individuals to meet their economic needs, such as employment or income. When these economic needs are met, patients are

BOX 3-1
Complex Communication Skills

I. **Contextual/Developmental Factors**
    Cultural issues in the interview
    Working with a translator
    Family interviewing
    The pediatric interview
    The adolescent interview
    The geriatric interview

II. **Assessment and Counseling**
    Smoking cessation
    Diet/exercise
    Cognitive dysfunction
    Risky sexual behaviors
    Anxiety/panic disorder
    Depressive disorders
    Domestic violence
    Alcoholism
    Drug addiction

III. **Challenging Situations**
    The angry patient/family
    Patients demanding inappropriate treatment
    Assessing and managing somatization and "problem patients"
    Discussing advanced directives
    Giving bad news
    Talking with patients about hospice care
    Talking with terminal patients about pain
    Being with a dying patient
    Talking with grieving patients/family members
    Talking to a patient/family about medical mistakes
    Terminating the doctor–patient relationship

IV. **Communicating with Colleagues**
    Communication with others on the health care team
    Talking to an impaired colleague
    Principles of teaching junior colleagues

less likely to have medical problems, are more likely to seek medical help, and are more likely to comply with medical interventions (IOM, 2003c).

Management of Difficult or Problematic Physician–Patient Interactions

Physicians consider about one in six patients in the outpatient care setting to be "difficult" (Hahn et al., 1996; Jackson and Kroenke, 1999). Such patients are not necessarily those with complex medical problems; rather, they are patients whom physicians perceive as being demanding and aggressive, seeking secondary gains, and/or having a variety of nonspecific complaints that persist despite the physician's best treatment efforts (Drossman, 1978; Novack and Landau, 1985; Steinmetz and Tabenkin, 2001). Difficult patients often have mental, mood, or personality disorders with or without comorbid alcohol abuse or dependence (Hahn et al., 1996; Jackson and Kroenke, 1999; Novack and Landau, 1985); display greater somatization (Jackson and Kroenke, 1999; Lin et al., 1991; Walker et al., 1997); and exhibit higher rates of health care utilization (Jackson and Kroenke, 1999; John et al., 1987; Lin et al., 1991). Problematic physician–patient interactions can result when patients with unmet expectations become dissatisfied with their care, and physicians become frustrated by patients who continue to complain despite the physician's therapeutic attempts (Jackson and Kroenke, 1999).

A number of investigators have recommended general treatment approaches for difficult patients that include treating the underlying issue, such as depression or somatization, and improving specific communication skills (Block and Coulehan, 1987; Drossman, 1978, 1997; Epstein et al., 1999; Katon et al., 1990; Kroenke and Swindle, 2000; Lidbeck, 2003; McLeod et al., 1997; Novack, 1993; Okugawa et al., 2002; Platt and Gordon, 1999; Quill, 1985, 1989; Schwenk and Romano, 1992; Smith, 1992). Students should be aware of these approaches. Additionally, educating students in how to work with difficult patients enhances their understanding of why the behavioral and social sciences are critical to their training. For example, physicians with positive attitudes toward psychosocial aspects of care may better recognize and empathize with the suffering of such patients (Cassell, 1999). Physicians with optimal communication skills that incorporate a biopsychosocial perspective may be less likely to label certain patients as difficult (Jackson and Kroenke, 1999; Levinson and Roter, 1995; Williamson et al., 1981), more likely to learn about and help alleviate such patients' emotional distress, and thereby engender greater patient satisfaction (Roter et al., 1995). Additionally, physicians with greater knowledge of the diagnosis of mental disorders are more likely to recognize and appropriately treat the mental health problems associated with difficult patients (Roter et al., 1997).

Medical students' success in working with difficult patients is related to the effectiveness of their instruction in the social and behavioral sciences. Students must have positive attitudes toward working with psychosocial aspects of care. They must also acquire effective interviewing skills that enable them to elicit and understand the multiple factors in patients' lives that may cause them to be difficult, including developmental issues such as deprivation and abuse, personality and affective disorders, substance abuse, and current life stressors. Students should know and be skillful in the therapeutic approaches that can be helpful to these patients.

SOCIAL AND CULTURAL ISSUES IN HEALTH CARE

High Priority

- Impact of social inequalities in health care and the social factors that are determinants of health outcomes
- Cultural competency

Medium Priority

- Role of complementary and alternative medicine

High-Priority Topics

Impact of Social Inequalities in Health Care and the Social Factors That Are Determinants of Health Outcomes

As emphasized throughout this report, the role of social factors in health outcomes is increasingly being recognized. It is now known more widely among researchers that morbidity, mortality, and disability rates have been linked to such social factors as race or ethnicity, education, income, and occupation. For example, African Americans and Native Americans consistently have among the worst disease outcomes, while Caucasian Americans typically survive disease with the best health outcomes. Both subtle and more blatant forms of discrimination have been documented in the U.S. health care system (Farley et al., 2001; Geiger and Borchelt, 2003; IOM, 2003c; Mayberry et al., 2000; Wojcik et al., 1998)—among different racial and ethnic groups, as well as between genders (Babey et al., 2003; Elster et al., 2003; Jha et al., 2003; Potosky et al., 2002).

Substantial evidence suggests that education and income are also linked to health outcomes. Those with higher socioeconomic status[3] fare the best, whereas those who are disadvantaged fare the worst (Kaplan and Keil, 1993; Kawachi and Kennedy, 1997; Marmot et al., 1991). The association between socioeconomic

---

[3]The committee recognizes that the terms *socioeconomic position* and *socioeconomic status* are both commonly used to describe a person's position in relation to social strata. For the sake of consistency, the committee uses the latter term in this report.

status and mortality is particularly striking because it appears to be graded and continuous. The finding that differences in health and mortality by socioeconomic status are not confined to those living in poverty or with poor access to health care indicates that other factors are also involved. Although there is clearly an inverse relationship between socioeconomic status and the prevalence of behaviors that pose a risk to health, statistical adjustment for behavioral and biological risk factors attenuates, but fails to eliminate, the excess mortality associated with low socioeconomic status (Davey Smith et al., 1998). Evidence suggests that contextual factors, such as poor social cohesion (Kawachi and Kennedy, 1997) and lack of community investment in human capital (Kaplan et al., 1996), are involved as well.

The workplace is another important social factor that can have adverse effects on health. Work conditions, including job demands, control, and latitude in decision making, have been found to be related to health outcomes (Karasek et al., 1988). Work-related stress, for example, has been associated with an increased incidence of coronary heart disease and a poorer prognosis in men with that condition (Schnall et al., 1994). Likewise, epidemiological studies have shown a relationship between downsizing or unemployment and cardiovascular disease risk (Mattiasson et al., 1990).

Medical students should be aware of the profound influence social factors can have on patients' health, including their health behaviors and outcomes. Students should be aware that they need to consider these factors if they are to provide optimal health care to all patients. Students should also understand the impact their social views can have on their ability to deliver effective health care.

Cultural Competency

Social factors such as those discussed above have also been found to influence how patients are treated by physicians (van Jaarsveld et al., 2001; van Ryn and Burke, 2000). The ability to understand and effectively treat diverse populations requires a recognition that the cultural context of illness can be an essential aspect of a successful therapeutic relationship (Braveman and Gruskin, 2003; Goodenough, 1981; IOM, 2003c). Culture, often in the form of ethnicity, provides a context for understanding normative beliefs and practices regarding health and illness (Dinan et al., 1991). For example, dementia is defined and perceived differently among various cultural groups (Bernstein et al., 2002; Dilworth-Anderson and Gibson, 2002; Henderson and Gutierrez-Mayka, 1992). Likewise, a survey of women of various races, cultures, geographic locations, and sexual orientations found that both decision-making patterns regarding certain female health issues and experiences with health care providers differed among the ethnic groups (Galavotti and Richter, 2000). African Americans expressed mistrust of physicians' motives for recommending a hysterectomy, as did several of the Caucasian, non-Hispanic women, whereas most of the Hispanic participants respected and trusted their providers. Interestingly, all the groups surveyed said they would seek additional medical opinions if they could afford to do so.

Careful attention to patients' language and language nuances offers a window into their cultural world view and explanatory models (Kleinman et al., 1978). Language nuances refer to how different cultural groups who speak the same language may use different phrases to refer to the same situation. Cultural nuances may be contextual, in that certain words are indigenous only to particular people within a certain region or locale. To avoid cultural stereotyping, it is vital for physicians to remember that there is wide intragroup diversity and that culture comes one patient at a time. This expression of culture at the individual level is referred to as "cultural frame," which is developed through the consolidation of the totality of one's experiences, interactions, and thoughts with the norms and expectations one perceives to be held by other members of a cultural group (Goodenough, 1981). Moreover, culture is expressed in many forms: ethnicity or national origin, religious traditions, regional norms and customs, occupational values and traditions, organizational norms, and geographic setting.

Medical students need to understand that cultural competency encompasses language, customs, values, belief systems, and rituals that patients bring to the medical encounter. Medical students, therefore, need to develop a level of cultural competency that moves them far beyond familiarity with a group to engender a firm understanding of how patients' language, customs, values, belief systems, and rituals can and do affect health care delivery, patient compliance, and effective and relevant doctor–patient communication.

Medium-Priority Topic

Role of Complementary and Alternative Medicine

People often seek health-related care from individuals other than biomedical practitioners (Foster and Anderson, 1978; NCCAM, 2003). A popular form of this practice is complementary and alternative medicine (CAM). Earlier as well as contemporary forms of CAM have been termed "folk medicine" and "medicine rooted in popular culture." Physicians often refer to themselves as "clinicians," whereas those practicing CAM therapy are considered "practitioners" (Sugarman and Burk, 1998), a distinction that invariably leads to stigmatization of CAM therapy as an ineffective method of treatment. It is important to recognize that many patients may be reticent to reveal their CAM-related beliefs and behaviors to their physicians, fearing disapproval or ridicule.

It has been estimated that 629 million visits were made to providers of CAM therapy in the United States in 1997 (Eisenberg et al., 1998), and in that same year, about 15 million U.S. adults were thought to have taken CAM therapy along with their prescription medications (Eisenberg et al., 1998). Medical students must be aware of and have knowledge of CAM practices, as recent studies have shown that a significant majority of people seeing a physician and using CAM therapies report preferring the use of both to the use of either alone (Astin, 1998; Eisenberg et al., 2001). Thus, medical students need to be skillful at eliciting information from their patients who are actively seeking or currently using other forms of treatment. Otherwise, patients may not disclose the other forms of care they use or their reasons for doing so.

Students should be encouraged to take an interest during regular office visits in their patients' rationale for using complementary, cultural, alternative, folk, or popular medicine. In addition, the content of medical school courses should include attention to those health-related practices that are unique to the region of the medical student's training (e.g., predominant ethnic and religious groups) and techniques for eliciting other treatments a patient may be undergoing. Rather than simply objecting to a patient who uses CAM, the medical student should consider the meaning a given practice may hold and the need it may meet—that is, the patient's view of its efficacy. At the same time, students need to be able to determine from a biomedical viewpoint whether a practice is helpful, harmful, or neutral. Given the possibility of severe drug interactions, all dietary supplements, medications, and nonprescription drugs being used by the patient should be ascertained when the history is taken (Piscitelli, 2000).

Additionally, patients may be turning to their physicians for guidance on whether these therapies are effective and safe and can be used concurrently with their prescription medications. Of the 117 medical schools responding to a 1997 survey, only 75 reported offering elective courses in CAM or including relevant CAM topics in required courses (Wetzel et al., 1998). Resistance to the incorporation of these therapies into medical education is the result of a common attitude that CAM therapies are not grounded in scientific method and are therefore not a priority in medical education (Sugarman and Burk, 1998; Wetzel et al., 2003). The most persuasive arguments for incorporating CAM into the curricula are made by recent studies showing the adverse effects of the use of CAM therapies concurrently with pharmaceuticals (Nortier et al., 2000; Piscitelli et al., 2000; Ruschitzka et al., 2000).

HEALTH POLICY AND ECONOMICS

High Priority

- Overview of U.S. health care system
- Economic incentives affecting patients' health-related behaviors
- Costs, cost-effectiveness, and physician responses to financial incentives

Medium Priority

- Variations in care

High-Priority Topics

Overview of U.S. Health Care System

Throughout their professional careers, physicians must make decisions about how to allocate scarce medical resources to improve health and satisfy wants. Health economics is the scientific study of these choices. In virtually all health care environments, physicians interact not only with patients, but also with insurers and myriad health care systems. Physicians trained in health economics—and health policy—will have a much better understanding of how resources should be allocated and what constraints are involved. The result will be better clinicians (Eisenberg, 1989a,b).

The undergraduate medical school curriculum provides the ideal opportunity for developing these foundations through basic instruction in health economics and health policy. This basic instruction should include, among other important topics, an overview of the U.S. health care system. Because this is such a broad subject, it is up to the individual medical school to determine the specific aspects of the system on which to focus.

One concept that might be addressed is that, unlike many other service sectors, the health care industry is dominated by the public sector. Public payments for health care services rose to $647 billion and paid almost half of all health care expenditures in 2001. Similarly, in just 30 years, the proportion of gross domestic product[4] spent on health care in the United States had doubled to roughly 14 percent by 2001 (Levit et al., 2003). Medical students can be taught to understand the unique role the U.S. health care industry plays in the larger economy and the trends that have motivated efforts to contain costs. This can be done by providing an overview of the U.S. health care system from the clinician's perspective. A

---

[4]Gross domestic product is a measure of the total goods and services produced at the national level.

good source is an article published by John Iglehart in the *New England Journal of Medicine* (Iglehart, 1998). It provides a basic understanding of the public and private insurance systems that is appropriate for medical students.

Students might also be taught that a broad cross section of Americans are uninsured (AHRQ, 2002), and that roughly one-quarter of the uninsured come from families with a member who has access to employer-provided insurance but chooses not to purchase it (Gruber and Washington, 2003). Such individuals may have access to free or subsidized care, but otherwise pay the full price of medical care from their own pockets and fail to benefit from the discounted fees and medication prices that health plans typically negotiate. Although many uninsured adults come from low-income households, some 19 percent of the uninsured are from families with incomes above 300 percent of the poverty line (Kaiser Family Foundation, 2003). The effects of being uninsured on health are the subject of ongoing study, with conflicting results (Bhattacharya et al., 2003; Goldman et al., 2001; Levy and Meltzer, 2001).

Medical students can be introduced to the different systems of care and their explicit (and implicit) attempts to control costs. Medicare and some Medicaid programs regulate the prices paid to providers directly. Capitated plans pay physicians a fixed amount regardless of how much care is delivered. Managed care plans sometimes intercede directly in the patient–provider relationship through practice guidelines, although physicians have chafed at the imposition of such controls (Studdert et al., 2002). In fact, most cost increases can be tied to the development of new medical technologies and the increased use of existing technologies. For example, increases in the supply of diagnostic imaging and cardiac, cancer, and neonatal technologies are associated with higher utilization and spending (Baker et al., 2003).

More generally, medical students can learn how medical services are rationed and how central their actions are to this process. As noted by Fuchs (1984), the basic method of rationing goods and services in this country is through the marketplace. The willingness of patients to purchase physician services and of physicians to supply them determines how they are apportioned and distributed.

For most nonmedical goods, consumers balance the benefits expected from a purchase against the cost, with the result being an efficient allocation of resources. Expenditures for medical services are different because most patients have insurance, and even the uninsured have a safety net. This means a third party is paying for care. The patient will therefore want additional care, and a "conscientious" physician will provide it even though its cost to society exceeds the benefit to the patient.

Regardless of the specific topics selected, medical students need to graduate with a basic understanding of the health care system that can be reinforced and further explored during postgraduate training.

Economic Incentives Affecting Patients' Health-Related Behaviors

Throughout their lives, patients make numerous complex decisions relating to their health. They engage in healthy (or risky) behaviors associated with diet, exercise, car safety, and smoking; they choose occupations and places to live that can place them in harm's way or expose them to deleterious environments. Medical students should have a conceptual understanding of how economic incentives shape healthy behaviors. Grossman (1972) provides an excellent model that can be used for this purpose. Grossman suggests that medical care can be viewed as one input into a "production function" that creates health. In this framework, health is a durable good in much the same way as education or a home. People make investments in their health, just as they invest in graduate-level education or new plumbing, for the purpose of realizing better outcomes in the future. The importance of this model lies in its predictive ability. The model explains why people (rationally) might have differing demands for health and, within a set of health care choices, might act on preferences that vary among individuals and/or among subpopulations. For example, a highly paid professional athlete may have more motivation to stay fit than an accountant. An understanding of this model would allow physicians to better predict patients' behaviors and to appreciate the limits on what medical care can do.

Grossman's model is an example of a broader set of "rational choice" models. Other rational choice or behavioral models may be more appropriate; what is important is that students understand the scientific underpinnings of the particular model being presented and not simply its application.

Costs, Cost-Effectiveness, and Physician Responses to Financial Incentives

Given the resource limitations noted above, it is not unethical to consider cost when providing patient care. In fact, the real cost of engaging in an activity is the benefit lost by not using the same resources for the most highly valued alternative. In the health care arena, cost-effectiveness is the formal study of the costs and benefits of a medical intervention to determine whether it is worth undertaking. Benefits are measured in terms of some standard clinical outcome, such as mortality rate, years of added life, or quality-adjusted life years. This is closely related to cost–benefit analysis, although in that case benefits are measured in monetary equivalents. Unfortunately, concepts such as cost-effectiveness are used in health care without an understanding of these formal methods, and misallocation of resources often results (Drummond et al., 1987). Eisenberg (1989b) provides a useful guide to the economic analysis of clinical practices. The goal is not to teach medical students to be analysts, but rather informed readers who can understand the usefulness and limitations of studies that use such terms as "cost-effective" in describing treatment options.

Medical students also should understand the role they will play in delivering services and affecting total costs. For example, physicians often prescribe additional treatments of little social benefit for insurance reasons. Insurance basically gives patients and their physicians incentives to use services until the marginal benefit of additional treatment is small, even though these services may be expensive for the insurer. The result is a loss to society (which is consuming services of limited benefit). Cost-containment efforts such as managed care generally—and practice guidelines in particular—can be viewed as a way to prevent this overuse and thereby improve quality of care.

These are only two examples of the many administrative mechanisms developed to control the overuse, and perhaps inappropriate use, of medical services by physicians and their patients. Such mechanisms also may include capitation versus fee-for-service differential payments for in-network versus out-of-network referrals, and withholding of payments subject to financial performance, quality, or patient satisfaction outcomes.

Medium-Priority Topic

Variations in Care

In 1938, Sir Allison Glover first presented a study documenting that the incidence of tonsillectomy varied dramatically and systematically by locale within the United Kingdom (Glover, 1938). Since then, an enormous body of medical literature has documented similar variations in treatment for numerous procedures across many similar locales. In their pioneering study, Wennberg and Gittelsohn (1973) found that the chance of receiving a tonsillectomy varied from 7 to 70 percent across similar towns in Vermont. Wennberg et al. (1987) compared the use of medical procedures in Boston and New Haven (two very similar cities in terms of the presence of major academic medical centers, demographics, incomes, and health insurance coverage rates), and found that Boston residents spent almost 87 percent more per capita than New Haven residents on hospital care. Medical students need to understand the traditional explanations for variations in practice patterns across geographic areas, including sampling variation, income, physician and hospital density, and underlying health status. Other economic explanations also need to be considered. In part, the variations in care may reflect the fact that even patients with identical diagnosis or symptoms may prefer different treatments. However, this heterogeneity means that doctors must help patients place a value on the risks associated with treatments and potential health outcomes.

4

Strategies for Incorporating the Behavioral and Social Sciences into Medical School Curricula

TASK 3: *Provide options for how changes in curricula can be achieved, such as encouraging the leadership of medical schools to incorporate behavioral and social sciences, funding opportunities that would advance this goal, or other novel approaches that would achieve this aim. In developing these options, the barriers to implementing curricula change and approaches to overcome these barriers should be considered.*

SUMMARY: *There are a number of barriers to the incorporation of behavioral and social science content into medical school curricula. Some of these barriers are common to medical school curriculum change in general, whereas others pertain more specifically to the behavioral and social sciences. These barriers include resistance from poorly informed faculty and administrators, inadequate resources to support faculty and curriculum development in the behavioral and social sciences, a lack of leadership, and dispersion of behavioral and social science faculty among multiple departments and other units.*

None of the barriers described in this chapter are insurmountable, however, and several strategies can be used to overcome them. For example, many medical schools lack faculty members who can serve as champions for the behavioral and social sciences in the curriculum. The committee believes this problem could be overcome by the creation of a career development award program. Such a program has been effective in other health-related disciplines. In the behavioral and social sciences, it could free recipients from other faculty responsibilities, permitting them to develop leadership skills, work toward improving the behavioral and social science content of the curriculum, and develop a research program in an area related to the behavioral and social sciences. Individuals receiving career development awards could be used as information resources by other schools trying to enhance the behavioral and social science content of their own curricula.

The committee also recommends the creation of a program that provides curriculum development awards. One major purpose of these awards would be to develop model behavioral and social science curricula that could be emulated at other schools. Another major purpose, of course, would be to improve the behavioral and social science curriculum at the school receiving the award. More specifically, such awards would provide medical schools with funds to improve the behavioral and social science content of their curricula and teaching techniques, as well as their assessment methodologies, which could include new assessment techniques in addition to multiple-choice questions. Curriculum development funds could also be used to improve the teaching and assessment skills of a broad range of faculty members involved in courses with content related to the behavioral and social sciences.

In addition to constituting an essential tool for measurement of an individual's ability to practice medicine, the U.S. Medical Licensing Examination (USMLE) exerts a major influence on medical school curricula because it indicates what subject matter licensing authorities believe is important. There is a lack of hard data regarding the proportion of the USMLE devoted to the behavioral and social sciences, but a number of knowledgeable individuals believe the percentage is inadequate and has decreased in recent years. The committee recommends that the National Board of Medical Examiners review the test items included on the USMLE to ensure that they adequately reflect the behavioral and social science subject matter recommended in Chapter 3 of this report.

Incorporation of the behavioral and social sciences into medical school curricula poses unique challenges to curriculum committees, especially when there is resistance from faculty and department chairs. Some faculty may be opposed because of a perception that the behavioral and social sciences are not "hard" sciences and are therefore somewhat less important than other topics in the curriculum. Other barriers include inadequate resources to support training of faculty leaders and curriculum development in the behavioral and social sciences. This chapter focuses on these barriers and strategies that can be used to overcome them.

It should be noted that, because there are limited published data on specific strategies for incorporating the behavioral and social sciences into medical school curricula, the committee found it necessary in developing such strategies to rely in part on more-generic studies related to medical school curriculum change, and in part on the collective experience of committee members and those interviewed during the course of this study.

It should also be noted that, while the committee makes suggestions and recommendations regarding both content and other ways to improve behavioral and social science instruction in medical school, the committee believes each school should design its own educational program, and has therefore not attempted to specify details of a behavioral and social science curriculum per se.

BARRIERS TO INCORPORATING THE BEHAVIORAL AND SOCIAL SCIENCES INTO MEDICAL SCHOOL CURRICULA

The development and administration of the medical school curriculum are the centralized responsibility of each school of medicine, but the curriculum is difficult to change, in part because so many individuals, departments, and committees are involved. Curriculum reform occurs when there is consensus or the need for change among faculty leaders (AAMC, 2000). At present, however, no consensus exists regarding the importance of the behavioral and social sciences in medical education, making curriculum committees uncertain about how to proceed.

A general lack of leadership in medical schools is often cited as the most fundamental barrier to curriculum change (Bland et al., 2000b).

Faculty and administrative leaders often oppose such change because they do not understand or agree with the vision and rationale for the change, are uncertain that the change will improve learning, are unwilling to undertake the extra work required during the planning process, or do not want to relinquish instructional time for something new. Resistance to change can also arise from faculty members' failure to understand the importance of content outside their own domains of knowledge, a lack of innovative teaching skills, and inadequate funding (Robins et al., 2000).

The behavioral and social sciences remain undiscovered by many medical school faculty members because they are not familiar with the literature and do not perceive these disciplines as relevant to the practice of medicine. Traditionally, "real medicine" has been defined exclusively as biological medicine—the domain of science—whereas the behavioral and social sciences are often referred to as "soft" sciences and are even considered by some to provide only marginal knowledge (Taylor, 2003a,b). Additional problems arise from a lack of available faculty with expertise in these areas. Not only do faculty members frequently lack the requisite knowledge, but they may also lack the pedagogical skills needed to capture student interest in these subjects (Beckman and Frankel, 1984; Benbassat et al., 2003; Freidin et al., 1990; Sachdeva, 2000). Moreover, it can be difficult for faculty to move from a traditional lecture format to small-group and problem-based learning formats, which are often more effective in teaching behavioral and social science content (see Chapter 2).

Resources for instruction in the behavioral and social sciences are often lacking, and it is rare that adequate funding is available to maintain a single departmental home for behavioral and social science faculty, who are often appointed to a variety of departments (e.g., medicine) or a research center. Two notable exceptions—the Department of Behavioral Science at the University of Kentucky College of Medicine, founded in 1959 (Strauss, 1996), and the Social Medicine Department at the University of North Carolina School of Medicine, established in 1978—have interdisciplinary faculty in their departments with joint appointments in their fields of expertise. The lack of a single home for behavioral and social science faculty is detrimental for two reasons: (1) diminished access to resources that typically flow through departments, and (2) the lack of a common ground for interaction among behavioral and social science faculty members.

Resources to support curriculum development and time for instruction in the behavioral and social sciences are often scarce. This is especially troublesome given that a successful behavioral and social science program requires additional resources to cover the cost of the many faculty needed to provide small-group instruction. The successful incorporation of the behavioral and social sciences into a medical school curriculum also requires central resources for faculty development (from the dean's office or the school of medicine) so that the new content and the process by which it is incorporated will be of high quality, and faculty will feel confident in educating students in these disciplines using new teaching methods.

In summary, curriculum development in the behavioral and social sciences often faces all of the barriers associated with institutional change in general in addition to the specific challenges associated with teaching these disciplines. Despite these and other barriers, however, the committee was able to identify successful efforts in major structural curriculum change in medical education that include the incorporation of behavioral and social science content into the curriculum.

STRATEGIES FOR CURRICULUM CHANGE

Medical school curricula undergo continual evaluation and updating as new scientific information becomes available, health care priorities change, and innovative instructional techniques are introduced. Although, as noted, there is relatively little information in the literature addressing the specific topic of curriculum development and change in relation to the behavioral and social sciences, there is considerable information regarding the characteristics of successful medical school curriculum change more generally. These characteristics include strong leadership, the presence of faculty development programs, a formal curriculum change process, curriculum development awards, and high-quality processes for assessment of student learning. These characteristics are discussed in turn below.

Strong Leadership

The presence of strong leadership is commonly cited as a primary factor in achieving successful curriculum change (AAMC, 2000; Bland et al., 2000b; Dannefer et al., 1998; Skochelak et al., 2001). Throughout the twentieth century, the most important experiments in curriculum change at U.S. medical schools were led by deans committed to educational reform (AAMC, 2000). Such strong leaders with a clear vision and effective communication skills are essential for all curriculum reform efforts.

Leaders can be found throughout medical schools. They include faculty members and administrators who provide direction to educational programs and mentor junior colleagues interested in teaching (Wilkerson and Irby, 1998). To achieve change, the dean and other key leaders need to articulate clearly their support for educational change and take concrete steps to address faculty concerns.

One way to recognize and encourage faculty able to take on leadership roles in curriculum reform is to establish a career development awards program. Investing in the careers of potential leaders in a discipline is a powerful and proven strategy for advancing that discipline (Gruppen et al., 2003). Such awards provide funds for a faculty member's time away from other commitments, allowing him or her to focus on developing leadership skills and ability, obtaining and refining relevant knowledge, designing educational methods, conducting relevant research, and designing curriculum. Award recipients may concentrate on one or two of these areas to develop expertise in the discipline at their institution and become the leader or champion of curriculum reform.

Faculty development and teaching scholar programs lasting a year or more have been successful in creating a cadre of educational leaders within a medical school (Gruppen et al., 2003; Steinert et al., 2003); however, there has been no such program for faculty in the behavioral and social sciences.

The career development award strategy can make it possible to reward scholarship in the teaching of the behavioral and social sciences and other activities that support learning in these disciplines.

Career development awards provide salary and other support for faculty members, allowing them to pursue the acquisition of new leadership skills, develop curriculum changes, or complete research projects. These awards have been used successfully to promote curriculum change and to enhance the careers of faculty in the pulmonary and cardiovascular sciences (ACS, 2003; NCI, 2000; NIH Guide, 2000; University of Wisconsin, 2003). Medical schools need to have a similar award system in the behavioral and social sciences to increase faculty knowledge in these disciplines and provide selected faculty the time and resources needed to develop behavioral and social science content, teaching methods, and evaluation strategies (Steinert et al., 2003). A well-supported career development program in the behavioral and social sciences would free promising faculty members from competing responsibilities so they could pursue such efforts. Individuals receiving the awards could also serve as resources for other medical schools trying to enhance their behavioral and social science curricula (Cooke et al., 2003; Morzinski and Simpson, 2003).

> **Conclusion 3.** *Instruction in the behavioral and social sciences suffers from a lack of qualified faculty, inadequate support and incentives for existing faculty, and the absence of career development programs in the behavioral and social sciences.*

> **Recommendation 3.** *Establish a career development award strategy.* **Because the provision of career development awards has been an effective strategy for improving instruction and research in other health-related areas, the Office of Behavioral and Social Sciences Research of the National Institutes of Health or private foundations, or both, should establish a career development awards program to produce leaders in the behavioral and social sciences in medical schools.**

Faculty Development Programs

In addition to developing a cadre of leaders in the behavioral and social sciences, there is a need to improve the behavioral and social science–related teaching skills of a broader group of medical school faculty. Faculty development leads to improved skills for all faculty members as educators and scholars, and should be part of institutional policies for the promotion of academic excellence (Wilkerson and Irby, 1998). The improved skills that can be achieved through faculty development include the ability to write educational objectives, design and select teaching methods, develop and apply principles of learning, have enhanced presentation skills, lead small-group discussions, use effective questioning strategies, refine evaluation and feedback skills, and use educational technologies effectively (Hemmer and Pangaro, 2000; Hewson, 2000; Lang et al., 2000; Neely et al., 2000; Sachdeva, 2000).

A curricular innovation is more likely to be adopted when the faculty members involved understand its theoretical underpinnings and are trained in the skills required for its implementation (Bland et al., 2000a). One initial training session for faculty at the beginning of a project is not enough. Follow-up coaching, coupled with opportunities to engage in problem solving with colleagues as new skills are being practiced, can significantly enhance the implementation process. Workshops lasting at least 2 days, followed up with practice, feedback, and reminders, have been found effective in changing teachers' knowledge, attitudes, and skills (Wilkerson and Irby, 1998).

Medical schools that have incorporated the behavioral and social sciences into their curricula have also provided instructional improvement grants designed to motivate faculty to work on targeted areas of curriculum management. Academies of medical educators at the University of California, San Francisco (UCSF) Medical School and Harvard Medical School are just two examples of this trend toward providing incentives for change. At Harvard, the academy provides direct support to a select group of faculty members for their talent in and dedication to education. This mechanism rewards teaching faculty, fosters educational innovation, and provides a forum for the exchange of ideas related to medical education that crosses departmental and institutional lines (Thibault et al., 2003). Similarly, the academy at UCSF fosters excellence in teaching by supporting and rewarding talented teachers (Cooke et al., 2003). Although neither program focuses solely on the behavioral and social sciences, the academy at UCSF has funded curriculum development in the behavioral and social sciences as part of its mini-grant program. In addition, UCSF initiated a mentoring program for junior faculty members built around peer observation of the junior faculty's teaching abilities, although this program is not directed at the behavioral and social sciences. When such a program is well organized, a positive association is found between participation in the program and career satisfaction in medical schools (Chew et al., 2003; Palepu et al., 1996; Pololi et al., 2002).

One high-priority area for faculty development that is especially important for the behavioral and social sciences is assessment (discussed more fully below). Medical educators should strongly consider increasing their faculty development efforts to improve the skills of their faculty in writing test questions in the behavioral and social sciences. Additionally, medical school faculty should be provided the resources and support needed to eliminate flawed multiple-choice questions from their tests (Downing, 2002a,b). To this end, faculty development should include not only training in how to write high-quality test questions in the behavioral and social sciences, but also feedback to the authors of those questions. Faculty development staff should include individuals who have been trained in test writing and measurement of student performance. Data derived from student feedback on the fairness of test questions can be used in the continuing dialogue between faculty development staff and the authors of the questions. Student assessment can also be improved through workshops that provide training in writing test questions. The National Board of Medical Examiners (NBME), for example, offers such workshops to help faculty construct better-quality multiple-choice questions in the basic and clinical sciences (NBME, 2003) and could serve as a similar resource for the writing of test questions in the behavioral and social sciences. Yet funds for faculty development to improve test-writing skills, and thus student assessment, continue to be scarce (Downing, 2002b).

Faculty development can also be designed to increase faculty members' basic understanding of the behavioral and social sciences, educate them on teaching techniques appropriate to those disciplines, and provide curriculum evaluation.

Formal Curriculum Change Process

Successful curriculum change processes have followed a standard model that includes needs assessment, specification of learning objectives, selection of content and teaching methods, and evaluation of the change.

Needs assessment involves determining the appropriateness of current curriculum content, teaching methods, and timing of instruction. Many medical schools have completed needs assessments of their curricula and have found gaps and redundancies. Some of the gaps consist of issues related to the behavioral and social sciences (AAMC, 2000). As a result, as noted earlier, medical training programs across the United States have begun to incorporate the behavioral and social sciences into their curricula (AAMC, 2000; Benbassat et al., 2003; Brook et al., 2000; Tang et al., 2002). Additionally, numerous schools have moved to adopt a more integrated curriculum after careful assessment, evaluation, and discussion of their current content and teaching methods (AAMC, 2000; Maizes et al., 2002; Robins et al., 2000; Stalburg and Stein, 2002; Stine et al., 2000; University of Rochester, 2002). The reason for this shift is that scientific investigation and health care practice increasingly require the integration of multiple disciplines to adequately represent new ways of thinking about human health and disease as a result of the emergence of molecular and cellular medicine (Irby and Hekelman, 1997; Tosteson, 1994)—reflecting the fact, noted earlier, that the structure of the medical school curriculum is adjusted in accordance with national changes in medical research and health care.

Once an initial needs assessment has been completed, the focus shifts to reaching agreement on learning objectives, identifying content, selecting teaching methods, and creating appropriate forms of assessment. In the case of the behavioral and social sciences, this process requires faculty members who can serve as theme coordinators or champions for the incorporation of these disciplines across the curriculum. Because the process involves curriculum committee reviews and negotiation with existing course directors so they will allow time for behavioral and social science content in their courses, interpersonal negotiation skills are helpful.

In an effort to improve an unpopular Medical Humanities course at Ohio State University, for example, just such a person was asked to take the lead. This champion initiated multiple changes that included converting the course into a case-based lecture with a small-group format and modifying the schedule from an all-day class to a 90-minute session every week over 2 years. He also identified the knowledge domains to be taught and the best ways to integrate the material into the curriculum, found module directors to take responsibility for each domain, formed a course committee, and recruited tutors for the small groups. As a result, many more students now attend the class than was the case when it was the Medical Humanities course (Doug Post, Ohio State University, personal communication, September 2003).

A critical component of any curriculum development project is its evaluation. A well-conducted evaluation serves to legitimize the innovation process, provides feedback to stakeholders, refines the program, and maintains faculty enthusiasm for the change (Bland et al., 2000b; Henry, 1996; Robins et al., 2000). The University of Rochester, for example, formally evaluates its fully integrated curriculum by examining data from the Association of American Medical Colleges' Graduation Questionnaire. The university also developed a questionnaire given to students at the end of years 1, 2, and 4 that addresses issues relevant to the behavioral and social sciences. This questionnaire includes student perceptions of how well the six curricular themes (many of which relate to the behavioral and social sciences) are taught. As another example, the Social Medicine Department at the University of North Carolina, Chapel Hill (UNC) evaluates its Medicine and Society course in two ways: (1) a centrally distributed course evaluation given to all students at the medical school, and (2) a customized evaluation designed by the Social Medicine Department to address its specific concerns. More empirically, a prospective pretest–posttest controlled trial—the strongest study design for determining the effect of a curriculum intervention (Campbell and Stanley, 1966; Fitz-Gibbon and Morris, 1987; Green, 2001)—has been used to evaluate the impact of education in the behavioral and social sciences on students' attitudes toward sociocultural issues in medicine (Tang et al., 2002).

Accurate evaluation of curriculum innovation requires time to assess important outcomes, which in some cases may necessitate separate funding dedicated to the completion of the evaluation (Wartman et al., 2001). In fact, any curriculum change effort comes at a cost. Acquiring the funds needed to launch the change may require the establishment of partnerships with external organizations, such as foundations, or the identification of internal sources of funding (Bland et al., 2000b). As the curriculum innovation progresses, care must be taken to ensure that sufficient funds are available to support the change effort so it can continue once the initial grant support has expired.

Evaluating the effectiveness and impact of the innovation can prove useful in leveraging funds for continuing the effort. In addition, funders should consider whether their support for curriculum innovations would have the most impact if directed toward specific departments or a more centralized source. For example, the Interdisciplinary Generalist Curriculum project of the federal Health Resources and Services Administration found that providing money to the dean's office was probably the best means of effecting a multidisciplinary curriculum change because the curriculum as a whole was affected, and centralized leadership was required.

Because curriculum change is a labor-intensive process, faculty members need protected time to plan activities associated with implementing and evaluating the reform. However, resources for this purpose are generally lacking (Griner and Danoff, 2000; IOM, 2001a; Meyer et al., 1997). This lack of resources is especially problematic for medical school faculty who want to work on incorporating the behavioral and social sciences into the curriculum, although exceptions do exist. For example, the Social Medicine Department at the UNC School of Medicine receives significant funding from the state legislature for medical education in the behavioral and social sciences, as well as dedicated federal resources through the Area Health Education Center Program. These direct-funding sources ensure the department's stability, setting it apart from departments at other medical schools that have cited major difficulties regarding the sustainability of their curricular changes in the behavioral and social sciences (Alan Cross, University of North Carolina; Jason Satterfield, UCSF; and Doug Post, Ohio State University, personal communication, September 2003). External funding does not, however, diminish the responsibility of medical schools to provide adequate internal support for the behavioral and social science program. Such support should include adequate core funding, an appropriate organizational "home" for the behavioral and social science faculty, and promotion and tenure criteria that reward accomplishments in the behavioral and social sciences as well as those in the traditional basic sciences and clinical disciplines.

Conclusion 4. *Financial support for efforts by U.S. medical schools to improve their curricular content, teaching methodologies, and assessment of student performance in the behavioral and social sciences is inadequate.*

Curriculum Development Awards

Whereas career development awards fund specific individuals, curriculum development awards fund schools to initiate or reform a curriculum. These resources go toward salary support for faculty members working on curriculum development, as well as administrative staff. The funds are often used to offer faculty development workshops that provide training in effective methods of teaching and assessing student competency.

The Health Resources and Services Administration has helped fund several curriculum development initiatives, including the Interdisciplinary Generalist Program, Undergraduate Medical Education for the 21st Century, and Women's Health in the Medical School Curriculum (HRSA, 2003; Rabinowitz et al., 2001). Similarly, the Nutrition Academic Award Program developed by the National Heart, Lung, and Blood Institute in 1997 awards 5-year grants to applicant U.S. medical schools to encourage the development or enhancement of medical school curricula (NHLBI, 2003c). Although these initiatives are excellent resources for curriculum reform that include components of the behavioral and social sciences, they are not specific to those disciplines.

Recommendation 4. *Establish curriculum development demonstration project awards.* **The National Institutes of Health or private foundations, or both, should establish a program that funds demonstration projects in behavioral and social science curriculum development at U.S. medical schools.**

Assessment of Student Learning

Assessment of individual students is an essential element of the instructional process, making it possible to determine the extent to which learning objectives have been met through a particular curriculum or instructional methodology (Blue et al., 2000). Assessment also focuses learners and program participants on the most important aspects of a program and often drives learning. Thus, it is important to consider all aspects of student assessment, from internal examinations within courses to external licensing examinations, to fully assess both students and the adequacy of the curriculum.

Most medical schools test their students throughout the curriculum using multiple-choice examinations with questions written by faculty members (Downing, 2002a; Jozefowicz et al., 2002). Although few studies evaluate the quality of these in-house examinations, a recent study from the NBME revealed that violations of the most basic item-writing principles are common in the achievement tests used in medical schools (Downing, 2002a; Jozefowicz et al., 2002). Poorly crafted test questions add an artificial layer of difficulty to examinations that can result in inflation or deflation of test scores (Downing, 2002a,b). Many faculty members simply do not have the psychometric expertise to write high-quality tests, a point that applies especially to faculty in the behavioral and social sciences, in which the content is often heavily contextual.

Multiple-choice questions are the most widely used format for knowledge assessment because, unlike open-ended questions, they allow for consistency in grading, a sampling of student knowledge in an area with vast amounts of information, and a cost-effective means of assessment. In addition, large numbers of examinations can be scored more easily, and the test is less time-consuming to administer (Anbar, 1991; Edelstein et al., 2000; Veloski et al., 1999). Nontraditional testing methods, however, such as short essay questions, structured oral examinations, and objective structured clinical examinations, may be better suited for use in the behavioral and social sciences because they reveal, more so than other modes of testing, how the student frames problems, appraises and replies to alternative views, evaluates evidence, and defends conclusions. As discussed above, regardless of the testing method used, it is critical that faculty development and assistance resources be provided to ensure that faculty produce high-quality evaluations of behavioral and social science content.

The material covered on the U.S. Medical Licensing Examination (USMLE) signals to teachers and students alike what is considered important in the field of medicine and thus what should be emphasized in medical school curricula (Elstein, 1993; Swanson et al., 1992). Despite considerable effort, the committee was unable to determine what proportion of the content of the exam is currently devoted to the behavioral and social sciences. In part this is due to the exam's integrative format and the emphasis NBME has placed on the presentation of material in a clinical context, since Step 1 of the USMLE replaced Part I of the NBME examination.[1] NBME also cites differences in defining what constitutes a behavioral and social science question as a factor in its inability to quantify behavioral and social science content on the exam (Gerry Dillon, NBME, personal communication, September 2003). It is the impression of a number of informed individuals, however, that the proportion of material on the USMLE devoted to the behavioral and social sciences has declined. Some believe this is due to changes in the overall design of the exam, while others cite difficulty in writing high-quality test questions on the part of experienced faculty who lack formal training in the behavioral and social sciences. The committee does not believe it is necessary to specify a particular number of behavioral and social science questions that should be on the exam. Rather, the designed questions, however many it may take, should sufficiently cover the topics delineated in this report. Likewise, the committee believes the behavioral and social sciences should be part of the new clinical skills exam that will soon be included as part of the USMLE series.

Conclusion 5. *The subject matter covered by questions on the U.S. Medical Licensing Examination has a significant impact on the curricular decisions made by U.S. medical schools. The committee believes that the U.S. Medical Licensing Examination currently places insufficient emphasis on test items related to the behavioral and social sciences.*

Recommendation 5. *Increase behavioral and social science content on the U.S. Medical Licensing Examination.* The National Board of Medical Examiners should review the test items included on the U.S. Medical Licensing Examination to ensure that it adequately reflects the topics in the behavioral and social sciences recommended in this report.

---

[1]Before the USMLE, NBME Part I was essentially a collection of seven independently developed tests in basic science areas. The behavioral sciences received equal coverage at that time.

References

AAMC (Association of American Medical Colleges). 1999a. *Curriculum Management and Evaluation: AAMC Curriculum Management & Information Tool (CurrMIT)*. [Online] Available: http://www.aamc.org/meded/curric/start.htm [accessed November 2003].

AAMC. 1999b. *Report III: Contemporary Issues in Medicine: Communication in Medicine. Medical School Objectives Project*. Washington, DC: Association of American Medical Colleges.

AAMC. 2000. *The Education of Medical Students: Ten Stories of Curriculum Change*. New York: Millbank Memorial Fund.

AAMC. 2003a. *Curriculum Directory*. [Online] Available: http://services.aamc.org/currdir/start.cfm [accessed September 2003].

AAMC. 2003b. *News from the AAMC*. [Online] Available: http://www.aamc.org [accessed October 2003].

AAMC. 2003c. *Medical School Graduation Questionnaire: All School Report 2002/2003*. Washington, DC: Division of Medical Education, American Association of Medical Schools.

AAMC. 2004. *CurrMIT Database*. Washington, DC: Association of American Medical Colleges.

ABIM (American Board of Internal Medicine). 2001. *American Board of Internal Medicine Home Page*. [Online] Available: http://www.abim.org/ [accessed November 2003].

ACS (American Cancer Society). 2003. *American Cancer Society Cancer Control Career Development Award for Primary Care Physicians: Policies*. Atlanta, GA: American Cancer Society, Inc., Extramural Grants Program.

AHRQ (Agency for Health Care Research and Quality). 2002. *Table 5. Health insurance coverage of the civilian noninstitutionalized population: Population estimates by type of coverage and selected population characteristics, United States, first half of 2002*. [Online] Available: http://www.meps.ahrq.gov/CompendiumTables/02Ch1/T5_E02.htm [accessed December 2003].

Alpert EJ. 1995. Violence in intimate relationships and the practicing internist: new "disease" or new agenda? *Annals of Internal Medicine*. 123(10): 774-781.

Anbar M. 1991. Comparing assessments of students' knowledge by computerized open-ended and multiple-choice tests. *Academic Medicine*. 66(7): 420-422.

Anderson NB, Scott PA. 1999. Making the case for psychophysiology during the era of molecular biology. *Psychophysiology*. 36(1): 1-13.

99

Anonymous. 1969. Self-awareness as a formal component of the curriculum. *Archives of Internal Medicine.* 124(3): 385-386.

Anonymous. 1988. World Conference on Medical Education of the World Federation for Medical Education: The Edinburgh Declaration. *Medical Education.* 22: 481-482.

Ashing-Giwa K. 1999. Health behavior change models and their socio-cultural relevance for breast cancer screening in African American women. *Women and Health.* 28(4): 53-71.

Astin JA. 1998. Why patients use alternative medicine: results of a national study. *Journal of the American Medical Association.* 279(19): 1548-1553.

Babey SH, Ponce NA, Etzioni DA, Spencer BA, Brown ER, Chawla N. 2003. Cancer screening in California: racial and ethnic disparities persist. Los Angeles: UCLA Center for Health Policy Research (PB2003-4): 1-6.

Bairey Merz CN, Dwyer J, Nordstrom CK, Walton KG, Salerno JW, Schneider RH. 2002. Psychosocial stress and cardiovascular disease: pathophysiological links. *Behavioral Medicine.* 27(4): 141-147.

Baker L, Birnbaum H, Geppert J, Mishol D, Moyneur E. 2003. The relationship between technology availability and health care spending. *Health Affairs: Web Exclusive.* [Online] Available: http://content.healthaffairs.org/cgi/reprint/hlthaff.w3.537v1 [accessed April 2004].

Baldwin PJ, Dodd M, Wrate RM. 1997a. Young doctors' health–I. How do working conditions affect attitudes, health and performance? *Social Science and Medicine.* 45(1): 35-40.

Baldwin PJ, Dodd M, Wrate RM. 1997b. Young doctors' health–II. Health and health behaviour. *Social Science and Medicine.* 45(1): 41-44.

The Balint Society. 2003. *Introduction.* [Online] Available: http://www.balint.co.uk/home.html [accessed November 2003].

Bandura A. 1986. *Social Foundations of Thought and Action: A Social Cognitive Theory.* Englewood Cliffs, NJ: Prentice-Hall.

Barefoot JC, Brummett BH, Helms MJ, Mark DB, Siegler IC, Williams RB. 2000. Depressive symptoms and survival of patients with coronary artery disease. *Psychosomatic Medicine.* 62(6): 790-795.

Barsky AJ, Borus JF. 1999. Functional somatic syndromes. *Annals of Internal Medicine.* 130(11): 910-921.

Barzansky B, Etzel SI. 2003. Educational programs in US medical schools, 2002-2003. *Journal of the American Medical Association.* 290(9): 1190-1196.

Beckman H, Markakis K, Suchman A, Frankel R. 1994. Getting the most from a 20-minute visit. *American Journal of Gastroenterology.* 89(5): 662-664.

Beckman HB, Frankel RM. 1984. The effect of physician behavior on the collection of data. *Annals of Internal Medicine.* 101(5): 692-696.

Ben-Eliyahu S, Yirmiya R, Liebeskind JC, Taylor AN, Gale RP. 1991. Stress increases metastatic spread of a mammary tumor in rats: evidence for mediation by the immune system. *Brain, Behavior, and Immunity.* 5(2): 193-205.

Ben-Nathan D, Feuerstein G. 1990. The influence of cold or isolation stress on resistance of mice to West Nile virus encephalitis. *Experientia.* 46(3): 285-290.

Ben-Nathan D, Lustig S, Danenberg HD. 1991. Stress-induced neuro-invasiveness of a neurovirulent noninvasive Sindbis virus in cold or isolation subjected mice. *Life Sciences.* 48(15): 1493-500.

Benbassat J, Baumal R, Borkan JM, Ber R. 2003. Overcoming barriers to teaching the behavioral and social sciences to medical students. *Academic Medicine.* 78(4): 372.

Bennett G. 1987. *The Wound and the Doctor: Healing, Technology and Power in Modern Medicine.* London: Secker and Warburg. Pp. 246-247.

Beresford SA, Curry SJ, Kristal AR, Lazovich D, Feng Z, Wagner EH. 1997. A dietary intervention in primary care practice: the Eating Patterns Study. *American Journal of Public Health.* 87(4): 610-616.

Bernstein CN, Frankenstein UN, Rawsthorne P, Pitz M, Summers R, McIntyre MC. 2002. Cortical mapping of visceral pain in patients with GI disorders using functional magnetic resonance imaging. *American Journal of Gastroenterology.* 97(2): 319-327.

Bhattacharya J, Goldman D, Sood N. 2003. The link between public and private insurance and HIV-related mortality. *Journal of Health Economics.* 22(6): 1105-1122.

Biondi M. 2001. *Effects of Stress on Immune Functions: An Overview.* 3rd edition. New York: Academic Press.

Black BP, Miles MS. 2002. Calculating the risks and benefits of disclosure in African American women who have HIV. *Journal of Obstetric, Gynecologic, and Neonatal Nursing.* 31(6): 688-697.

Bland CJ, Starnaman S, Harris D, Henry R, Hembroff L. 2000a. "No fear" curricular change: monitoring curricular change in the W.K. Kellogg Foundation's National Initiative on Community Partnerships and Health Professions Education. *Academic Medicine.* 75(6): 623-633.

Bland CJ, Starnaman S, Wersal L, Moorehead-Rosenberg L, Zonia S, Henry R. 2000b. Curricular change in medical schools: how to succeed. *Academic Medicine.* 75(6): 575-594.

Block MR, Coulehan JL. 1987. Teaching the difficult interview in a required course on medical interviewing. *Journal of Medical Education.* 62(1): 35-40.

Blue AV, Barnette JJ, Ferguson KJ, Garr DR. 2000. Evaluation methods for prevention education. *Academic Medicine.* 75(7 Suppl): S28-S34.

Boelen C. 1995. Prospects for change in medical education in the twenty-first century. *Academic Medicine.* 70(7 Suppl): S21-S28; discussion S29-S31.

Bolman WM. 1995. The place of behavioral science in medical education and practice. *Academic Medicine.* 70(10): 873-878.

Bonneau RH, Sheridan JF, Feng NG, Glaser R. 1991. Stress-induced suppression of herpes simplex virus (HSV)-specific cytotoxic T lymphocyte and natural killer cell activity and enhancement of acute pathogenesis following local HSV infection. *Brain, Behavior, and Immunity.* 5(2): 170-192.

Bourgeois JA, Kay J, Rudisill JR, Bienenfeld D, Gillig P, Klykylo WM, Markert RJ. 1993. Medical student abuse: perceptions and experience. *Medical Education.* 27(4): 363-370.

Boyd MD, Weinrich SP, Weinrich M, Norton A. 2001. Obstacles to prostate cancer screening in African-American men. *Journal of National Black Nurses Association.* 12(2): 1-5.

Branch WT Jr, Kern D, Haidet P, Weissmann P, Gracey CF, Mitchell G, Inui T. 2001. The patient-physician relationship. Teaching the human dimensions of care in clinical settings. *Journal of the American Medical Association.* 286(9): 1067-1074.

Brashear DB. 1987. Support groups and other supportive efforts in residency programs. *Journal of Medical Education.* 62(5): 418-424.

Braveman P, Gruskin S. 2003. Defining equity in health. *Journal of Epidemiology and Community Health.* 57(4): 254-258.

Bridges KW, Goldberg DP. 1985. Somatic presentation of DSM III psychiatric disorders in primary care. *Journal of Psychosomatic Research.* 29(6): 563-569.

Brook DW, Gordon C, Meadow H, Cohen MC. 2000. Behavioral medicine in medical education: report of a survey. *Social Work in Health Care.* 31(2): 15-29.

Brook DW, Brook JS, Rosen Z, De La Rosa M, Montoya ID, Whiteman M. 2003. Early risk factors for violence in Colombian adolescents. *American Journal of Psychiatry.* 160(8): 1470-1478.

Burke BL, Arkowitz H, Menchola M. 2003. The efficacy of motivational interviewing: a meta-analysis of controlled clinical trials. *Journal of Consulting and Clinical Psychology.* 71(5): 843-861.

Byrne N, Wasylenki D. 1996. Developing a social contract between the medical school and the community. *Israel Journal of Medical Sciences.* 32(3-4): 222-228.

Campbell DT, Stanley, JC. 1966. *Experimental and Quasi-Experimental Designs for Research.* Chicago: Rand McNally.

Carmel S. 1997. The professional self-esteem of physicians scale, structure, properties, and the relationship to work outcomes and life satisfaction. *Psychological Reports*. 80(2): 591-602.

Carpenter S. 2001. Curriculum overhaul gives behavioral medicine a higher profile. *Monitor on Psychology*. 32(10).

Carr JE. 1998. Proposal for and integrated science curriculum in medical education. *Teaching and Learning in Medicine*. 10(1): 3-7.

Carroll BJ, Curtis GC, Davies BM, Mendels J, Sugerman AA. 1976. Urinary free cortisol excretion in depression. *Psychological Medicine*. 6(1): 43-50.

Cassano P, Fava M. 2002. Depression and public health: an overview. *Journal of Psychosomatic Research*. 53(4): 849-857.

Cassell EJ. 1999. Diagnosing suffering: a perspective. *Annals of Internal Medicine*. 131(7): 531-534.

CDC (Centers for Disease Control and Prevention). 1999. Tobacco use—United States, 1900–1999. *Morbidity and Mortality Weekly Report*. 48(43): 986–993.

CDC. 2002a. *Deaths—Leading Causes for 2000*. Atlanta, GA: National Center for Health Statistics.

CDC. 2002b. Trends in sexual risk behaviors among high school students—United States, 1991–2001. *Morbidity and Mortality Weekly Report*. 51(38): 856-9.

CDC. 2003. *Table 10. Estimated numbers of persons living with AIDS, by year and selected characteristics, 1998–2002—United States*. [Online] Available: http://www.cdc.gov/hiv/stats/hasr1402/table10.htm [accessed November 2003].

Chang PP, Ford DE, Mead LA, Cooper-Patrick L, Klag MJ. 1997. Insomnia in young men and subsequent depression. The Johns Hopkins Precursors Study. *American Journal of Epidemiology*. 146(2): 105-114.

Charmandari E, Kino T, Souvatzoglou E, Chrousos GP. 2003. Pediatric stress: hormonal mediators and human development. *Hormone Research*. 59(4): 161-179.

Cheng TL, DeWitt TG, Savageau JA, O'Connor KG. 1999. Determinants of counseling in primary care pediatric practice: physician attitudes about time, money, and health issues. *Archives of Pediatrics and Adolescent Medicine*. 153(6): 629-635.

Chew LD, Watanabe JM, Buchwald D, Lessler DS. 2003. Junior faculty's perspectives on mentoring. *Academic Medicine*. 78(6): 652.

Christ GH. 2000. Impact of development on children's mourning. *Cancer Practice*. 8(2): 72-81.

Christie-Seely JE. 1986. A diagnostic problem and family assessment. *Journal of Family Practice*. 22(4): 329-333, 337-339.

Ciechanowski PS, Katon WJ, Russo JE. 2000. Depression and diabetes: impact of depressive symptoms on adherence, function, and costs. *Archives of Internal Medicine*. 160(21): 3278-3285.

Clark DC, Zeldow PB. 1988. Vicissitudes of depressed mood during four years of medical school. *Journal of the American Medical Association*. 260(17): 2521-2528.

Clark DC, Salazar-Grueso E, Grabler P, Fawcett J. 1984. Predictors of depression during the first 6 months of internship. *American Journal of Psychiatry*. 141(9): 1095-1098.

Cleeland CS. 1998. Undertreatment of cancer pain in elderly patients. *Journal of the American Medical Association*. 279(23): 1914-1915.

Cleeland CS, Gonin R, Baez L, Loehrer P, Pandya KJ. 1997. Pain and treatment of pain in minority patients with cancer. The Eastern Cooperative Oncology Group Minority Outpatient Pain Study. *Annals of Internal Medicine*. 127(9): 813-816.

Clever LH. 2001. A checklist for making good choices in trying- or tranquil-times. *Western Journal of Medicine*. 174(1): 41-43.

Cochran N, Schiffman J. 2003. *New Directions 216: On Doctoring-Year 2*. [Online] Available: http://www.dartmouth.edu/dms/ed_programs/courses/courses_yr2_ondoctoring.shtml [accessed August 2003].

Cohen S. 1995. Psychological stress and susceptibility to upper respiratory infections. *American Journal of Respiratory and Critical Care Medicine*. 152(4 Pt 2): S53-S58.

Cole SA, Bird J. 2000. *The Medical Interview*. 2nd edition. St. Louis: Mosby, Inc.

Cooke M, Irby DM, Debas HT. 2003. The UCSF Academy of Medical Educators. *Academic Medicine*. 78(7): 666-672.

Coombs RH, Virshup BB. 1994. Enhancing the psychological health of medical students: the student well-being committee. *Medical Education*. 28(1): 47-54, discussion 55-57.

Coulehan J, Belling C, Williams PC, McCrary SV, Vetrano M. 2003. Human contexts: medicine in society at Stony Brook University School of Medicine. *Academic Medicine*. 78(10): 987-992.

Coulehan JL, Block MR. 2001. *The Medical Interview*. Philadelphia: F.A. Davis Co.

Craig AD. 2003. Pain mechanisms: labeled lines versus convergence in central processing. *Annual Review of Neuroscience*. 26: 1-30.

Crawley LM, Marshall PA, Lo B, Koenig BA. 2002. Strategies for culturally effective end-of-life care. *Annals of Internal Medicine*. 136(9): 673-679.

Dannefer EF, Johnston MA, Krackov SK. 1998. Communication and the process of educational change. *Academic Medicine*. 73(9 Suppl): S16-S23.

Davey Smith G, Neaton JD, Wentworth D, Stamler R, Stamler J. 1998. Mortality differences between black and white men in the USA: contribution of income and other risk factors among men screened for the MRFIT. MRFIT Research Group. Multiple Risk Factor Intervention Trial. *Lancet*. 351(9107): 934-939.

Dhabhar FS, McEwen BS. 1999. Enhancing versus suppressive effects of stress hormones on skin immune function. *Proceedings of the National Academy of Sciences of the United States of America*. 96(3): 1059-1064.

Dickstein LH. 2001. Educating for professionalism: creating a culture of humanism in medical education. *Journal of the American Medical Association*. 285(24): 3147-3148.

Dilworth-Anderson P, Gibson BE. 2002. The cultural influence of values, norms, meanings, and perceptions in understanding dementia in ethnic minorities. *Alzheimer Disease and Associated Disorders*. 16(Suppl 2): S56-S63.

DiMatteo MR. 1994a. Enhancing patient adherence to medical recommendations. *Journal of the American Medical Association*. 271(1): 79, 83.

DiMatteo MR. 1994b. The physician-patient relationship: effects on the quality of health care. *Clinical Obstetrics and Gynecology*. 37(1): 149-161.

Dinan TG, O'Keane V, O'Boyle C, Chua A, Keeling PW. 1991. A comparison of the mental status, personality profiles and life events of patients with irritable bowel syndrome and peptic ulcer disease. *Acta Psychiatrica Scandinavica*. 84(1): 26-28.

Dismuke SE, McClary AM. 2000. Putting it all together: building a four-year curriculum. *Academic Medicine*. 75(7 Suppl): S90-S92.

Downing SM. 2002a. Threats to the validity of locally developed multiple-choice tests in medical education: construct-irrelevant variance and construct underrepresentation. *Advances in Health Sciences Education: Theory and Practice*. 7(3): 235-241.

Downing SM. 2002b. Construct-irrelevant variance and flawed test questions: do multiple-choice item-writing principles make any difference? *Academic Medicine*. 77(10 Suppl): S103-S104.

Drexel University. 2003. [Online] Available: http://webcampus.med.drexel.edu/admissions/curriculum.asp [accessed November 2003].

Drossman DA. 1978. The problem patient. Evaluation and care of medical patients with psychosocial disturbances. *Annals of Internal Medicine*. 88(3): 366-372.

Drossman DA. 1997. Psychosocial sound bites: exercises in the patient-doctor relationship. *American Journal of Gastroenterology*. 92(9): 1418-1423.

Drummond M, Stoddart G, Labelle R, Cushman R. 1987. Health economics: an introduction for clinicians. *Annals of Internal Medicine*. 107(1): 88-92.

Dube CE, O'Donnell JF, Novack DH. 2000. Communication skills for preventive interventions. *Academic Medicine*. 75(7 Suppl): S45-S54.

Edelstein RA, Reid HM, Usatine R, Wilkes MS. 2000. A comparative study of measures to evaluate medical students' performance. *Academic Medicine*. 75(8): 825-833.

Eisenberg DM, Davis RB, Ettner SL, Appel S, Wilkey S, Van Rompay M, Kessler RC. 1998. Trends in alternative medicine use in the United States, 1990-1997: results of a follow-up national survey. *Journal of the American Medical Association.* 280(18): 1569-1575.

Eisenberg DM, Kessler RC, Van Rompay MI, Kaptchuk TJ, Wilkey SA, Appel S, Davis RB. 2001. Perceptions about complementary therapies relative to conventional therapies among adults who use both: results from a national survey. *Annals of Internal Medicine.* 135(5): 344-531.

Eisenberg JM. 1989a. How can we pay for graduate medical education in ambulatory care? *New England Journal of Medicine.* 320(23): 1525-1531.

Eisenberg JM. 1989b. Clinical economics: a guide to the economic analysis of clinical practices. *Journal of the American Medical Association.* 262(20): 2879-2886.

Elstein AS. 1993. Beyond multiple-choice questions and essays: the need for a new way to assess clinical competence. *Academic Medicine.* 68(4): 244-249.

Elster A, Jarosik J, VanGeest J, Fleming M. 2003. Racial and ethnic disparities in health care for adolescents: a systematic review of the literature. *Archives of Pediatrics and Adolescent Medicine.* 157(9): 867-874.

Ely JW, Goerdt CJ, Bergus GR, West CP, Dawson JD, Doebbeling BN. 1998. The effect of physician characteristics on compliance with adult preventive care guidelines. *Family Medicine.* 30(1): 34-39.

Engel GL. 1977. The need for a new medical model: a challenge for biomedicine. *Science.* 196(4286): 129-136.

Epstein RM. 1999. Mindful practice. *Journal of the American Medical Association.* 282(9): 833-839.

Epstein RM, Campbell TL, Cohen-Cole SA, McWhinney IR, Smilkstein G. 1993. Perspectives on patient-doctor communication. *Journal of Family Practice.* 37(4): 377-388.

Epstein RM, Quill TE, McWhinney IR. 1999. Somatization reconsidered: incorporating the patient's experience of illness. *Archives of Internal Medicine.* 159(3): 215-222.

Epstein RM, Dannefer EF, Nofziger AC, Hansen JT, Schultz SH, Jospe N, Connard LW, Meldrum SC, Henson LC. In Press. Comprehensive assessment of professional competence: the Rochester experiment. *Teaching and Learning in Medicine.* 16(2).

Evans RG, Stoddart GL. 1990. Producing health, consuming health care. *Social Science and Medicine.* 31(12): 1347-1363.

Everson SA, Goldberg DE, Kaplan GA, Cohen RD, Pukkala E, Tuomilehto J, Salonen JT. 1996. Hopelessness and risk of mortality and incidence of myocardial infarction and cancer. *Psychosomatic Medicine.* 58(2): 113-121.

Fang WL, Applegate SN, Stein RM, Lohr JA. 1998. The development of substance-abuse curricular content by five North Carolina schools. *Academic Medicine.* 73(10): 1039-1043.

Farkas AJ, Pierce JP, Zhu SH, Rosbrook B, Gilpin EA, Berry C, Kaplan RM. 1996. Addiction versus stages of change models in predicting smoking cessation. *Addiction.* 91(9): 1271-1280, discussion 1281-1292.

Farley JH, Hines JF, Taylor RR, Carlson JW, Parker MF, Kost ER, Rogers SJ, Harrison TA, Macri CI, Parham GP. 2001. Equal care ensures equal survival for African-American women with cervical carcinoma. *Cancer.* 91(4): 869-873.

Faulkner LR, McCurdy RL. 2000. Teaching medical students social responsibility: the right thing to do. *Academic Medicine.* 75(4): 346-350.

Fields AI, Cuerdon TT, Brasseux CO, Getson PR, Thompson AE, Orlowski JP, Youngner SJ. 1995. Physician burnout in pediatric critical care medicine. *Critical Care Medicine.* 23(8): 1425-1429.

Fields SA, Toffler WL, Elliott D, Chappelle K. 1998. Principles of clinical medicine: Oregon Health Sciences University School of Medicine. *Academic Medicine.* 73(1): 25-31.

Fiore M, Bailey W, Cohen S, Dorfman S, Goldstein M, Gritz E, Heyman R, Jaen C, Kottke T, Lando H, Mecklenburg R, Mullen P, Nett L, Robinson L, Stitzer M, Tomasello A, Villejo L, Wewers M. 2000. *Treating Tobacco Use and Dependence, Clinical Practice Guideline.* Rockville, MD: U.S. Department of Health and Human Services.

Firth-Cozens J. 2001. Interventions to improve physicians' well-being and patient care. *Social Science and Medicine*. 52(2): 215-222.

Fitz-Gibbon CT, Morris LL. 1987. How to design a program evaluation (book number 3). In: *Program Evaluation Kit*. Newbury Park, CA: Sage.

Fletcher RH, Fletcher SW, Wagner EH. 1998. *Clinical Epidemiology: The Essentials*. 3rd edition. Philadelphia: Lippincott, Williams, and Wilkins.

Flexner A. 1910. *Medical Education in the United States and Canada*. Boston: Merrymount Press.

Foster GM, Anderson BG. 1978. *Medical Anthropology*. New York: Wiley.

Frasure-Smith N, Lesperance F, Talajic M. 1993. Depression following myocardial infarction. Impact on 6-month survival. *Journal of the American Medical Association*. 270(15): 1819-1825.

Freidin RB, Goldman L, Cecil RR. 1990. Patient-physician concordance in problem identification in the primary care setting. *Annals of Internal Medicine*. 93(3): 490-493.

Frelix GD, Rosenblatt R, Solomon M, Vikram B. 1999. Breast cancer screening in underserved women in the Bronx. *Journal of the National Medical Association*. 91(4): 195-200.

Freund KM, Bak SM, Blackhall L. 1996. Identifying domestic violence in primary care practice. *Journal of General Internal Medicine*. 11(1): 44-46.

Friedman M, Thoresen CE, Gill JJ, Ulmer D, Powell LH, Price VA, Brown B, Thompson L, Rabin DD, Breall WS, Bourg W, Levy R, Dieon T. 1986. Alteration of type A behavior and its effect on cardiac recurrences in post myocardial infarction patients: summary results of the recurrent coronary prevention project. *American Heart Journal*. 112(4): 653-665.

Friedman SB, Ader R, Glasgow LA. 1965. Effects of psychological stress in adult mice inoculated with Coxsackie B Virus. *Psychosomatic Medicine*. 27: 361-368.

Fuchs VR. 1984. The "rationing" of medical care. *New England Journal of Medicine*. 311(24): 1572-1573.

Gabbard GO, Menninger RW. 1989. The psychology of postponement in the medical marriage. *Journal of the American Medical Association*. 261(16): 2378-2381.

Galavotti C, Richter DL. 2000. Talking about hysterectomy: the experiences of women from four cultural groups. *Journal of Women's Health and Gender-Based Medicine*. 9(Suppl 2): S63-S67.

Galianti G. 1997. *Caring for Patients from Different Cultures*. Philadelphia: University of Pennsylvania Press.

Geiger HJ, Borchelt G. 2003. Racial and ethnic disparities in US health care. *Lancet*. 362(9396): 1674.

Geurts S, Rutte C, Peeters M. 1999. Antecedents and consequences of work-home interference among medical residents. *Social Science and Medicine*. 48(9): 1135-1148.

Gin NE, Rucker L, Frayne S, Cygan R, Hubbell FA. 1991. Prevalence of domestic violence among patients in three ambulatory care internal medicine clinics. *Journal of General Internal Medicine*. 6(4): 317-322.

Glasgow RE, Strycker LA, Toobert DJ, Eakin E. 2000. A social-ecologic approach to assessing support for disease self-management: the Chronic Illness Resources Survey. *Journal of Behavioral Medicine*. 23(6): 559-583.

Glasgow RE, Hiss RG, Anderson RM, Friedman NM, Hayward RA, Marrero DG, Taylor CB, Vinicor F. 2001a. Report of the health care delivery work group: behavioral research related to the establishment of a chronic disease model for diabetes care. *Diabetes Care*. 24(1): 124-130.

Glasgow RE, Orleans CT, Wagner EH. 2001b. Does the chronic care model serve also as a template for improving prevention? *Milbank Quarterly*. 79(4): 579-612, iv-v.

Glasgow RE, Funnell MM, Bonomi AE, Davis C, Beckham V, Wagner EH. 2002. Self-management aspects of the improving chronic illness care breakthrough series: implementation with diabetes and heart failure teams. *Annals of Behavioral Medicine*. 24(2): 80-87.

Glover A. 1938. The incidence of tonsillectomy in school children. *Proceedings of the Royal Society of Medicine*. 31: 1219-1236.

Goldberg EL, Van Natta P, Comstock GW. 1985. Depressive symptoms, social networks and social support of elderly women. *American Journal of Epidemiology.* 121(3): 448-456.

Goldberg RJ, Novack DH. 1992. The psychosocial review of systems. *Social Science and Medicine.* 35(3): 261-269.

Goldberg RJ, Novack DH, Gask L. 1992. The recognition and management of somatization: what is needed in primary care training. *Psychosomatics.* 33(1): 55-61.

Goldman DP, Bhattacharya J, Leibowitz AA, Joyce GF, Shapiro MF, Bozzette SA. 2001. The impact of state policy on the costs of HIV infection. *Medical Care Research and Review.* 58(1): 31-53, discussion 54-59.

Goldstein MG, Ruggiero L, Guise BJ, Abrams DB. 1994. Behavioral medicine strategies for medical patients. In: Stoudemire A, Ed. *Clinical Psychiatry for Medical Students.* 2nd edition. Philadelphia: J.B. Lippincott Co. Pp. 671-693.

Goldstein MG, DePue J, Kazura A, Niaura R. 1998. Models for provider-patient interaction: applications to health behavior change. In: Shumaker SA, Schron J, Ockene M, Eds. *Handbook of Health Behavior Change.* 2nd edition. New York: Springer-Verlag. Pp. 85-113.

Goodenough WH. 1981. *Culture, Language, and Society.* Menlo Park, CA: Benjamin Cummings Publishing.

Gorlin R, Zucker HD. 1983. Physicians' reactions to patients. A key to teaching humanistic medicine. *New England Journal of Medicine.* 308(18): 1059-1063.

Graves KD, Miller PM. 2003. Behavioral medicine in the prevention and treatment of cardiovascular disease. *Behavior Modification.* 27(1): 3-25.

Green ML. 2001. Identifying, appraising, and implementing medical education curricula: a guide for medical educators. *Annals of Internal Medicine.* 135(10): 889-896.

Griner PF, Danoff D. 2000. Sustaining change in medical education. *Journal of the American Medical Association.* 283(18): 2429-2431.

Grossman M. 1972. On the concept of health capital and the demand for health. *The Journal of Political Economy.* 80(2): 223-255.

Gruber J, Washington E. 2003. *Subsidies to Employee Health Insurance Premiums and the Health Insurance Market.* NBER Working Paper Series. Cambridge, MA: National Bureau of Economic Research.

Grueninger U, Duffy F, Goldstein M. 1995. Patient education in the medical encounter: how to facilitate learning, behavior change and coping. In: Lipkin MJ, Putnam S, Lazare A, Eds. *The Medical Interview: Clinical Care, Education, Research.* New York: Springer-Verlag. Pp. 122-133.

Gruppen LD, Woolliscroft JO, Wolf FM. 1988. The contribution of different components of the clinical encounter in generating and eliminating diagnostic hypotheses. *Proceedings of the Annual Conference on Research in Medical Education.* 27: 242-247.

Gruppen LD, Frohna AZ, Anderson RM, Lowe KD. 2003. Faculty development for educational leadership and scholarship. *Academic Medicine.* 78(2): 137-141.

Hahn RA, Teutsch SM, Rothenberg RB, Marks JS. 1990. Excess deaths from nine chronic diseases in the United States, 1986. *Journal of the American Medical Association.* 264(20): 2654-2659.

Hahn SR, Thompson KS, Wills TA, Stern V, Budner NS. 1994. The difficult doctor-patient relationship: somatization, personality and psychopathology. *Journal of Clinical Epidemiology.* 47(6): 647-657.

Hahn SR, Kroenke K, Spitzer RL, Brody D, Williams JB, Linzer M, deGruy FV 3rd. 1996. The difficult patient: prevalence, psychopathology, and functional impairment. *Journal of General Internal Medicine.* 11(1): 1-8.

Haidet P, Paterniti DA. 2003. "Building" a history rather than "taking" one: a perspective on information sharing during the medical interview. *Archives of Internal Medicine.* 163(10): 1134-1140.

Hamberger LK, Saunders DG, Hovey M. 1992. Prevalence of domestic violence in community practice and rate of physician inquiry. *Family Medicine.* 24(4): 283-287.

HBCC (Health and Behavior Coordinating Committee). 1993. *NIH Implementation Plan for Health and Behavior Research: Report to Congress.* Bethesda, MD: NIH Office of Disease Prevention.

Hemmer PA, Pangaro L. 2000. Using formal evaluation sessions for case-based faculty development during clinical clerkships. *Academic Medicine.* 75(12): 1216-1221.

Henderson JN, Gutierrez-Mayka M. 1992. Ethnocultural themes in caregiving to Alzheimer's disease patients in Hispanic families. *Clinical Gerontologist.* 11: 59-74.

Hendrie HC, Clair DK, Brittain HM, Fadul PE. 1990. A study of anxiety/depressive symptoms of medical students, house staff, and their spouses/partners. *Journal of Nervous and Mental Disease.* 178(3): 204-207.

Henry RC. 1996. Evaluation as a tool for reform. In: Richards RW, Ed. *Building Partnerships: Educating Health Professionals for the Communities They Serve.* San Francisco, CA: Jossey-Bass.

Hertzman C, Power C. 2003. Health and human development: understandings from life-course research. *Developmental Neuropsychology.* 24(2-3): 719-744.

Hewson MG. 2000. A theory-based faculty development program for clinician-educators. *Academic Medicine.* 75(5): 498-501.

Holtzman D, Powell-Griner E, Bolen JC, Rhodes L. 2000. State- and sex-specific prevalence of selected characteristics—Behavioral Risk Factor Surveillance System, 1996 and 1997. *MMWR CDC Surveillance Summaries.* 49(6): 1-39.

Hoyert DL. 1996. *Medical and Life-Style Risk Factors Affecting Fetal Mortality, 1989-1990: Vital Health Statistics.* Hyattsville, MD: National Center for Health Statistics.

HRSA (Health Resources and Services Administration). 2003. *Women's Health in the Medical School Curriculum.* [Online] Available: http:www.hrsa.gov/WomensHealth/medschl.htm [accessed December 2003].

Ickovics JR, Hamburger ME, Vlahov D, Schoenbaum EE, Schuman P, Boland RJ, Moore J. 2001. Mortality, CD4 cell count decline, and depressive symptoms among HIV-seropositive women: longitudinal analysis from the HIV Epidemiology Research Study. *Journal of the American Medical Association.* 285(11): 1466-1474.

Iglehart JK. 1998. Medicare and graduate medical education. *New England Journal of Medicine.* 338(6): 402-407.

IIME (The Institute for International Medical Education). 2003. *The IIME.* [Online] Available: http://www.iime.org/iime.htm [accessed October 2003].

IOM (Institute of Medicine). 1983. *Medical Education and Societal Needs: A Planning Report for Health Professions.* Washington, DC: National Academy Press.

IOM. 2000. *Promoting Health: Intervention Strategies from Social and Behavioral Research.* Smedley BD, Syme SL, Eds. Washington, DC: National Academy Press.

IOM. 2001a. *Crossing the Quality Chasm: A New Health System for the 21st Century.* Washington, DC: National Academy Press.

IOM. 2001b. *Health and Behavior: The Interplay of Biological, Behavioral, and Societal Influences.* Washington, DC: National Academy Press.

IOM. 2003a. *Health Professions Education: A Bridge to Quality.* Washington, DC: The National Academies Press.

IOM. 2003b. *Microbial Threats to Health: Emergence, Detection, and Response.* Washington, DC: The National Academies Press.

IOM. 2003c. *Unequal Treatment: Confronting Racial and Ethnic Disparities in Health Care.* Washington, DC: The National Academies Press.

Irby DM, Hekelman FP. 1997. Future directions for research on faculty development. *Family Medicine.* 29(4): 287-289.

Jackson JL, Kroenke K. 1999. Difficult patient encounters in the ambulatory clinic: clinical predictors and outcomes. *Archives of Internal Medicine.* 159(10): 1069-1075.

Januzzi JL Jr, Stern TA, Pasternak RC, DeSantis RW. 2000. The influence of anxiety and depression on outcomes of patients with coronary artery disease. *Archives of Internal Medicine.* 160(13): 1913-1921.

Jha AK, Varosy PD, Kanaya AM, Hunninghake DB, Hlatky MA, Waters DD, Furberg CD, Shlipak MG. 2003. Differences in medical care and disease outcomes among black and white women with heart disease. *Circulation.* 108(9): 1089-1094.

John C, Schwenk TL, Roi LD, Cohen M. 1987. Medical care and demographic characteristics of "difficult" patients. *Journal of Family Practice.* 24(6): 607-610.

Jozefowicz RF, Koeppen BM, Case S, Galbraith R, Swanson D, Glew RH. 2002. The quality of in-house medical school examinations. *Academic Medicine.* 77(2): 156-161.

Kadushin G. 2000. Family secrets: disclosure of HIV status among gay men with HIV/AIDS to the family of origin. *Social Work in Health Care.* 30(3): 1-17.

Kahn GS, Cohen B, Jason H. 1979. The teaching of interpersonal skills in U.S. medical schools. *Journal of Medical Education.* 54(1): 29-35.

Kaiser Family Foundation. 2003. *The Uninsured: A Primer.* Washington, DC: The Henry J. Kaiser Family Foundation.

Kalichman SC, DiMarco M, Austin J, Luke W, DiFonzo K. 2003. Stress, social support, and HIV-status disclosure to family and friends among HIV-positive men and women. *Journal of Behavioral Medicine.* 26(4): 315-332.

Kann L, Warren CW, Harris WA, Collins JL, Williams BI, Ross JG, Kolbe LJ. 1996. Youth Risk Behavior Surveillance—United States, 1995. *MMWR CDC Surveillance Summaries.* 45(4): 1-84.

Kaplan GA, Keil JE. 1993. Socioeconomic factors and cardiovascular disease: a review of the literature. *Circulation.* 88(4 Pt 1): 1973-1998.

Kaplan GA, Pamuk ER, Lynch JW, Cohen RD, Balfour JL. 1996. Inequality in income and mortality in the United States: analysis of mortality and potential pathways. *British Medical Journal.* 312(7037): 999-1003.

Kaplan HI, Sadock B, Grebb JA. 1994. *Kaplan and Sadock's Synopsis of Psychiatry.* 7th edition. Baltimore, MD: Williams and Wilkens.

Karasek RA, Theorell T, Schwartz JE, Schnall PL, Pieper CF, Michela JL. 1988. Job characteristics in relation to the prevalence of myocardial infarction in the US Health Examination Survey (HES) and the Health and Nutrition Examination Survey (HANES). *American Journal of Public Health.* 78(8): 910-918.

Katon W. 1984. Depression: relationship to somatization and chronic medical illness. *Journal of Clinical Psychiatry.* 45(3 Pt 2): 4-12.

Katon W, Russo J. 1989. Somatic symptoms and depression. *Journal of Family Practice.* 29(1): 65-69.

Katon W, Von Korff M, Lin E, Lipscomb P, Russo J, Wagner E, Polk E. 1990. Distressed high utilizers of medical care: DSM-III-R diagnoses and treatment needs. *General Hospital Psychiatry.* 12(6): 355-362.

Kawachi I, Kennedy BP. 1997. Health and social cohesion: why care about income inequality? *British Medical Journal.* 314(7086): 1037-1040.

Kawachi I, Colditz GA, Ascherio A, Rimm EB, Giovannucci E, Stampfer MJ, Willett WC. 1996. A prospective study of social networks in relation to total mortality and cardiovascular disease in men in the USA. *Journal of Epidemiology and Community Health.* 50(3): 245-251.

Keller CS, Allan JD. 2001. Evaluation of selected behavior change theoretical models used in weight management interventions. *Online Journal of Knowledge Synthesis for Nursing.* 8: 5.

Kellner R. 1990. Somatization: theories and research. *Journal of Nervous and Mental Disease.* 178(3): 150-160.

King S, Dixon MJ. 1996. The influence of expressed emotion, family dynamics, and symptom type on the social adjustment of schizophrenic young adults. *Archives of General Psychiatry.* 53(12): 1098-1104.

Kleinman A, Eisenberg L, Good B. 1978. Culture, illness, and care: clinical lessons from anthropologic and cross-cultural research. *Annals of Internal Medicine.* 88(2): 251-258.

Krantz DS, Santiago HT, Kop WJ, Bairey Merz CN, Rozanski A, Gottdiener JS. 1999. Prognostic value of mental stress testing in coronary artery disease. *American Journal of Cardiology.* 84(11): 1292-1297.

Krantz G, Ostergren PO. 2000. Common symptoms in middle aged women: their relation to employment status, psychosocial work conditions and social support in a Swedish setting. *Journal of Epidemiology and Community Health.* 54(3): 192-199.

Kripke EN, Steele G, O'Brien MK, Novack DH. 1998. Domestic violence training program for residents. *Journal of General Internal Medicine.* 13(12): 839-841.

Kroenke K. 1992. Symptoms in medical patients: an untended field. *American Journal of Medicine.* 92(1A): 3S-6S.

Kroenke K. 2003. Patients presenting with somatic complaints: epidemiology, psychiatric comorbidity and management. *International Journal of Methods in Psychiatric Research.* 12(1): 34-43.

Kroenke K, Swindle R. 2000. Cognitive-behavioral therapy for somatization and symptom syndromes: a critical review of controlled clinical trials. *Psychotherapy and Psychosomatics.* 69(4): 205-215.

Kroenke K, Spitzer RL, Williams JB, Linzer M, Hahn SR, deGruy FV 3rd, Brody D. 1994. Physical symptoms in primary care: predictors of psychiatric disorders and functional impairment. *Archives of Family Medicine.* 3(9): 774-779.

Kurtz S, Silverman J, Draper J. 1998. *Teaching and Learning Communication Skills in Medicine.* Abington, Oxon, UK: Radcliffe Medical Press.

Lang F, Everett K, McGowen R, Bennard B. 2000. Faculty development in communication skills instruction: insights from a longitudinal program with "real-time feedback". *Academic Medicine.* 75(12): 1222-1228.

Lazare A, Putnam SM, Lipkin M Jr. 1995. Three functions of the medical interview. In: Lipkin M Jr, Putnam SM, Lazare A, Eds. *The Medical Interview.* New York: Springer-Verlag. Pp. 3-19.

LCME (Liaison Committee on Medical Education). 2003. *Functions and Structure of a Medical School: Standards for Accreditation of Medical Education Programs Leading to the M.D. Degree.* Washington, DC: Liaison Committee on Medical Education.

Lee Y, Choi K, Lee YK. 2001. Association of comorbidity with depressive symptoms in community-dwelling older persons. *Gerontology.* 47(5): 254-262.

Leserman J, Drossman DA. 1995. Sexual and physical abuse history and medical practice. *General Hospital Psychiatry.* 17(2): 71-74.

Leserman J, Li Z, Hu YJ, Drossman DA. 1998. How multiple types of stressors impact on health. *Psychosomatic Medicine.* 60(2): 175-181.

Leserman J, Petitto JM, Golden RN, Gaynes BN, Gu H, Perkins DO, Silva SG, Folds JD, Evans DL. 2000. Impact of stressful life events, depression, social support, coping, and cortisol on progression to AIDS. *American Journal of Psychiatry.* 157(8): 1221-1228.

Levinson W, Roter D. 1995. Physicians' psychosocial beliefs correlate with their patient communication skills. *Journal of General Internal Medicine.* 10(7): 375-379.

Levinson W, Gorawara-Bhat R, Lamb J. 2000. A study of patient clues and physician responses in primary care and surgical settings. *Journal of the American Medical Association.* 284(8): 1021-1027.

Levit K, Smith C, Cowan C, Lazenby H, Sensenig A, Catlin A. 2003. Trends in U.S. health care spending, 2001. *Health Affairs.* 22(1): 154-164.

Levy H, Meltzer D. 2001. *What Do We Really Know About Whether Health Insurance Affects Health?* Chicago: University of Chicago, Harris Graduate School of Public Policy Studies.

Lidbeck J. 2003. Group therapy for somatization disorders in primary care: maintenance of treatment goals of short cognitive-behavioural treatment one-and-a-half-year follow-up. *Acta Psychiatrica Scandinavica.* 107(6): 449-456.

Lin EH, Katon W, Von Korff M, Bush T, Lipscomb P, Russo J, Wagner E. 1991. Frustrating patients: physician and patient perspectives among distressed high users of medical services. *Journal of General Internal Medicine.* 6(3): 241-246.

Linzer M, Visser MR, Oort FJ, Smets EM, McMurray JE, de Haes HC. 2001. Predicting and preventing physician burnout: results from the United States and the Netherlands. *American Journal of Medicine.* 111(2): 170-175.

Lipkin M Jr, Frankel RM, Beckman HB, Charon R, Fein O. 1995a. Performing the interview. In: Lipkin M Jr, Putnam SM, Lazare A, Eds. *The Medical Interview.* New York: Springer-Verlag. Pp. 65-82.

Lipkin M Jr, Kaplan C, Clark W, Novack DH. 1995b. Teaching medical interviewing: The Lipkin Model. In: Lipkin M Jr, Putnam SM, Lazare A, Eds. *The Medical Interview: Clinical Care, Education and Research.* New York: Springer-Verlag. Pp. 422-435.

Longhurst M. 1988. Physician self-awareness: the neglected insight. *Canadian Medical Association Journal.* 139(2): 121-124.

Luban PB. 1995. Empowerment techniques: from doctor-centered (Balint Approach) to patient-centered discussion groups. *Patient Education and Counseling.* 26: 257-263.

Lubitz RM, Nguyen DD. 1996. Medical student abuse during third-year clerkships. *Journal of the American Medical Association.* 275(5): 414-416.

Ludmerer KM. 1985. *Learning to Heal: The Development of American Medical Education.* New York: Basic Books Inc.

Ludmerer KM. 1999. *Time to Heal: American Medical Education from the Turn of the Century to the Era of Managed Care.* New York: Oxford University Press.

Lustman PJ, Clouse RE, Freedland KE. 1998. Management of major depression in adults with diabetes: implications of recent clinical trials. *Seminars in Clinical Neuropsychiatry.* 3(2): 102-114.

Maekawa SJ, Aoyama N, Shirasaka D, Kuroda K, Tamura T, Kuroda Y, Kasuga M. 2003. Excessive alcohol intake enhances the development of synchronous cancerous lesion in colorectal cancer patients. *International Journal of Colorectal Disease.* 19(2): 171-175.

Maizes V, Schneider C, Bell I, Weil A. 2002. Integrative medical education: development and implementation of a comprehensive curriculum at the University of Arizona. *Academic Medicine.* 77(9): 851-860.

Makoul G. 1998. Communication research in medical education. In: Jackson L, Duffy B, Eds. *Health Communication Research: A Guide to Developments and Directions.* Westport, CT: Greenwood Press. Pp. 17-35.

Makoul G, Curry RH, Novack DH. 1998. The future of medical school courses in professional skills and perspectives. *Academic Medicine.* 73(1): 48-51.

Marmot MG, Smith GD, Stansfeld S, Patel C, North F, Head J, White I, Brunner E, Feeney A. 1991. Health inequalities among British civil servants: the Whitehall II study. *Lancet.* 337(8754): 1387-1393.

Marshall AA, Smith RC. 1995. Physicians' emotional reactions to patients: recognizing and managing countertransference. *American Journal of Gastroenterology.* 90(1): 4-8.

Martin AR. 1986. Stress in residency: a challenge to personal growth. *Journal of General Internal Medicine.* 1(4): 252-257.

Marvel MK, Epstein RM, Flowers K, Beckman HB. 1999. Soliciting the patient's agenda: have we improved? *Journal of the American Medical Association.* 281(3): 283-287.

Matthews DA, Suchman AL, Branch WT Jr. 1993. Making "connexions": enhancing the therapeutic potential of patient-clinician relationships. *Annals of Internal Medicine.* 118(12): 973-977.

Mattiasson I, Lindgarde F, Nilsson JA, Theorell T. 1990. Threat of unemployment and cardiovascular risk factors: longitudinal study of quality of sleep and serum cholesterol concentrations in men threatened with redundancy. *British Medical Journal.* 301(6750): 461-466.

Mayberry RM, Mili F, Ofili E. 2000. Racial and ethnic differences in access to medical care. *Medical Care Research and Review.* 57(Suppl 1): 108-145.

Mayne TJ, Vittinghoff E, Chesney MA, Barrett DC, Coates TJ. 1996. Depressive affect and survival among gay and bisexual men infected with HIV. *Archives of Internal Medicine.* 156(19): 2233-2238.

McCoy CB, Smith SA, Metsch LR, Anwyl RS, Correa R, Bankston L, Zavertnik JJ. 1994. Breast cancer screening of the medically underserved: results and implications. *Cancer Practice.* 2(4): 267-274.

McCranie EW, Brandsma JM. 1988. Personality antecedents of burnout among middle-aged physicians. *Behavioral Medicine.* 14(1): 30-36.

McCurdy L, Goode LD, Inui TS, Daugherty RM Jr, Wilson DE, Wallace AG, Weinstein BM, Copeland EM 3rd. 1997. Fulfilling the social contract between medical schools and the public. *Academic Medicine.* 72(12): 1063-1070.

McEwen BS. 2002. Sex, stress and the hippocampus: allostasis, allostatic load and the aging process. *Neurobiology of Aging.* 23(5): 921-939.

McGinnis JM, Foege WH. 1993. Actual causes of death in the United States. *Journal of the American Medical Association.* 270(18): 2207-2212.

McKegney CP. 1989. Medical education: a neglectful and abusive family system. *Family Medicine.* 21(6): 452-457.

McLeod CC, Budd MA, McClelland DC. 1997. Treatment of somatization in primary care. *General Hospital Psychiatry.* 19(4): 251-258.

Melzack R, Wall PD. 1965. Pain mechanisms: a new theory. *Science.* 150(699): 971-979.

Mendes de Leon CF, Powell LH, Kaplan BH. 1991. Change in coronary-prone behaviors in the recurrent coronary prevention project. *Psychosomatic Medicine.* 53(4): 407-419.

Meyer GS, Potter A, Gary N. 1997. A national survey to define a new core curriculum to prepare physicians for managed care practice. *Academic Medicine.* 72(8): 669-676.

Milan FB, Goldstein MG, Novack DH, O'Brien MK. 1998. Are medical schools neglecting clinical skills? A survey of U.S. medical schools. *Annals of Behavioral Science and Medical Education.* 5(1): 3-12.

Miller WR, Rollnick S. 2002. *Motivational Interviewing: Preparing People to Change Addictive Behavior.* 2nd edition. New York: Guilford.

Minino AM, Arias E, Kochanek KD, Murphy SL, Smith BL. 2002. *National Vital Statistics Reports (NVSS). Deaths: Final Data for 2000.* Hyattsville, MD: National Center for Health Statistics. Vol 50.

Mokdad AH, Marks JS, Stroup DF, Gerberding JL. 2004. Actual causes of death in the United States, 2000. *Journal of American Medical Association.* 291(10): 1238-1245.

Montgomery V, Oliver R, Reisner A, Fallat ME. 2002. The effect of severe traumatic brain injury on the family. *Journal of Trauma.* 52(6): 1121-1124.

Morsiani M, Beretta P, Pareschi PL, Manservigi D, Bottoni L. 1985. Long-term results in preventive medicine for type II diabetes. *Acta Diabetologica Latina.* 22(3): 191-202.

Morzinski JA, Simpson DE. 2003. Outcomes of a comprehensive faculty development program for local, full-time faculty. *Family Medicine.* 35(6): 434-9.

Muller S. 1984. Physicians for the twenty-first century: report of the project panel on the general professional education of the physician and college preparation for medicine. *Journal of Medical Education.* 59(11 Part 2).

Myers MF. 2001. The well-being of physician relationships. *Western Journal of Medicine.* 174(1): 30-33.

Nanchahal K, Ashton WD, Wood DA. 2000. Alcohol consumption, metabolic cardiovascular risk factors and hypertension in women. *International Journal of Epidemiology.* 29(1): 57-64.

Nawaz H, Adams ML, Katz DL. 2000. Physician-patient interactions regarding diet, exercise, and smoking. *Preventive Medicine.* 31(6): 652-657.

NBME (National Board of Medical Examiners). 2003. *Services for Medical Schools.* [Online] Available: http://www.nbme.org/programs/medsch.asp [accessed August 2003].

NCCAM (National Center for Complementary and Alternative Medicine). 2003. *NCCAM Home.* [Online] Available: http://nccam.nih.gov [accessed October 2003].

NCHS (National Center for Health Statistics). 2002. *Health, United States: 2002: Table 67*. Hyattsville, MD: Centers for Disease Control and Prevention.

NCHS. 2003a. *Health, United States, 2003: With Chartbook on Trends in the Health of Americans*. Hyattsville, MD: Centers for Disease Control and Prevention.

NCHS. 2003b. *National Vital Statistics Reports: Deaths: Final Data for 2001*. Hyattsville, MD: Centers for Disease Control and Prevention.

NCI (National Cancer Institute). 2000. *Career Development and Training Program for Basic Scientists*. [Online] Available: http://www3.cancer.gov/bip/trngscitst.htm [accessed October 2003].

NCME (Northwest Center for Medical Education). 2003. *Step 3: Systemic Function*. [Online] Available: http://shaw.medlib.iupui.edu/nwcme/nwcme.html [accessed November 2003].

Neely KL, Stifel EN, Milberg LC. 2000. A systematic approach to faculty development in women's health: lessons from education, feminism, and conflict theory. *Academic Medicine*. 75(11): 1095-1101.

NHLBI (National Heart, Lung, and Blood Institute). 2003a. *Chronic Obstructive Pulmonary Disease*. Bethesda, MD: National Institutes of Health, National Heart, Lung, and Blood Institute.

NHLBI. 2003b. *Coronary Heart Disease*. Bethesda, MD: National Institutes of Health, National, Heart, Lung, and Blood Institute.

NHLBI. 2003c. *NAA National Site at the National Heart, Lung, and Blood Institute*. [Online] Available: http://www.nhlbi.nih.gov/funding/training/naa/ [accessed October 2003].

NIAAA (National Institute on Alcohol Abuse and Alcoholism). 1998. *Alcohol Alert No. 42: Alcohol and the Liver, Research Update*. Rockville, MD: National Institute on Alcohol Abuse and Alcoholism.

NIAAA. 2002. *Alcohol: What You Don't Know Can Harm You*. Rockville, MD: National Institutes of Health.

Nightingale SD, Yarnold PR, Greenberg MS. 1991. Sympathy, empathy, and physician resource utilization. *Journal of General Internal Medicine*. 6: 420-442.

NIH Guide. 2000. *Academic Career Award (K07)*. [Online] Available: http://grants1.nih.gov/grants/guide/pa-files/PA-00-070.html [accessed October 2003].

Nortier JL, Martinez MC, Schmeiser HH, Bieler CA, Petein M, Depierreux MF, De Pauw L, Abramowicz D, Vereerstraeten P, Vanherweghem JL. 2000. Urothelial carcinoma associated with the use of a Chinese herb (Aristolochia fangchi). *New England Journal of Medicine*. 342(23): 1686-1692.

Novack DH. 1987. Therapeutic aspects of the clinical encounter. *Journal of General Internal Medicine*. 2(5): 346-355.

Novack DH. 1993. Active management of problem patients. *British Journal of Hospital Medicine*. 50(10): 573-574, 576.

Novack DH. 1998. Communication challenges. *Medical Encounter*. 14: 25.

Novack DH, Landau C. 1985. Psychiatric diagnoses in problem patients. *Psychosomatics*. 26(11): 853-855, 858.

Novack DH, Volk G, Drossman DA, Lipkin M Jr. 1993. Medical interviewing and interpersonal skills teaching in US medical schools. Progress, problems, and promise. *Journal of the American Medical Association*. 269(16): 2101-2105.

Novack DH, Suchman AL, Clark W, Epstein RM, Najberg E, Kaplan C. 1997. Calibrating the physician. Personal awareness and effective patient care. Working Group on Promoting Physician Personal Awareness, American Academy on Physician and Patient. *Journal of the American Medical Association*. 278(6): 502-509.

Novack DH, Epstein RM, Paulsen RH. 1999. Toward creating physician-healers: fostering medical students' self-awareness, personal growth, and well-being. *Academic Medicine*. 74(5): 516-520.

NRC (National Research Council). 2001. *New Horizons in Health: An Integrative Approach*. Singer BH, Ryff CD, Eds. Washington, DC: National Academy Press.

O'Loughlin J, Makni H, Tremblay M, Lacroix C, Gervais A, Dery V, Meshefedjian G, Paradis G. 2001. Smoking cessation counseling practices of general practitioners in Montreal. *Preventive Medicine.* 33(6): 627-638.

Ohio State University. 2003. [Online] Available: http://medicine.osu.edu/futurestudents/curriculum_blueprint.cfm [accessed November 2003].

Okugawa G, Yagi A, Kusaka H, Kinoshita T. 2002. Paroxetine for treatment of somatization disorder. *Journal of Neuropsychiatry and Clinical Neurosciences.* 14(4): 464-465.

Orth-Gomer K, Rosengren A, Wilhelmsen L. 1993. Lack of social support and incidence of coronary heart disease in middle-aged Swedish men. *Psychosomatic Medicine.* 55(1): 37-43.

Osler W, Harvey AM. 1976. *The Principles and Practice of Medicine.* 19th edition. New York: Appleton-Century-Crofts and Fleschner Pub. Co.

Palan BM, Chandwani S. 1989. Coping with examination stress through hypnosis: an experimental study. *American Journal of Clinical Hypnosis.* 31(3): 173-80.

Palepu A, Friedman RH, Barnett RC. 1996. Medical faculty with mentors are more satisfied. *Journal of General Internal Medicine.* 11(Suppl): 5107.

Papadakis MA, Osborn EH, Cooke M, Healy K. 1999. A strategy for the detection and evaluation of unprofessional behavior in medical students. University of California, San Francisco School of Medicine Clinical Clerkships Operation Committee. *Academic Medicine.* 74(9): 980-990.

Parboosingh J. 2003. Medical schools' social contract: more than just education and research. *Canadian Medical Association Journal.* 168(7): 852-853.

Partnership for Solutions. 2003. *Latest Additions.* [Online] Available: http://www.partnershipforsolutions.org/ [accessed October 2003].

Paxton S. 2000. Public disclosure of serostatus—the impact on HIV-positive people. *Sex Health Exchange.* (1): 13-14.

Pessione F, Ramond MJ, Peters L, Pham BN, Batel P, Rueff B, Valla DC. 2003. Five-year survival predictive factors in patients with excessive alcohol intake and cirrhosis. Effect of alcoholic hepatitis, smoking and abstinence. *Liver International.* 23(1): 45-53.

Peters AS, Greenberger-Rosovsky R, Crowder C, Block SD, Moore GT. 2000. Long-term outcomes of the New Pathway Program at Harvard Medical School: a randomized controlled trial. *Academic Medicine.* 75(5): 470-479.

Peterson MC, Holbrook JH, Von Hales D, Smith NL, Staker LV. 1992. Contributions of the history, physical examination, and laboratory investigation in making medical diagnoses. *Western Journal of Medicine.* 156(2): 163-165.

Pettus MC. 2002. Implementing a medicine-spirituality curriculum in a community-based internal medicine residency program. *Academic Medicine.* 77(7): 745.

Pilowsky I. 1988. An outline curriculum on pain for medical schools. *Pain.* 33(1): 1-2.

Piscitelli S. 2000. Preventing dangerous drug interactions. *Journal of the American Pharmaceutical Association.* 40(5 Suppl 1): S44-S45.

Piscitelli SC, Burstein AH, Chaitt D, Alfaro RM, Falloon J. 2000. Indinavir concentrations and St. John's wort. *Lancet.* 355(9203): 547-548.

Platt FW, Gordon GH. 1999. *Field Guide to the Difficult Patient Interview.* Baltimore, MD: Lippincott Williams & Wilkens.

Platt FW, Platt CM. 2003. Two collaborating artists produce a work of art: the medical interview. *Archives of Internal Medicine.* 163(10): 1131-1132 .

Platt FW, Gaspar DL, Coulehan JL, Fox L, Adler AJ, Weston WW, Smith RC, Stewart M. 2001. "Tell me about yourself": the patient-centered interview. *Annals of Internal Medicine.* 134(11): 1079-1085.

Pololi LH, Knight SM, Dennis K, Frankel RM. 2002. Helping medical school faculty realize their dreams: an innovative, collaborative mentoring program. *Academic Medicine.* 77(5): 377-384.

Portenoy RK, Lesage P. 1999. Management of cancer pain. *Lancet.* 353(9165): 1695-1700.

Potosky AL, Harlan LC, Kaplan RS, Johnson KA, Lynch CF. 2002. Age, sex, and racial differences in the use of standard adjuvant therapy for colorectal cancer. *Journal of Clinical Oncology.* 20(5): 1192-1202.

Power C, Hertzman C. 1997. Social and biological pathways linking early life and adult disease. *British Medical Bulletin.* 53(1): 210-221.

Prochaska JO, DiClemente CC. 1986. Towards a comprehensive model of change. In: Miller WR, Heather N, Eds. *Treating Addictive Disorders: Processes of Change.* New York: Plenum Press.

Quill TE. 1985. Somatization disorder: one of medicine's blind spots. *Journal of the American Medical Association.* 254(21): 3075-3079.

Quill TE. 1989. Recognizing and adjusting to barriers in doctor-patient communication. *Annals of Internal Medicine.* 111(1): 51-57.

Quill TE, Williamson PR. 1990. Healthy approaches to physician stress. *Archives of Internal Medicine.* 150(9): 1857-1861.

Rabinowitz HK, Babbott D, Bastacky S, Pascoe JM, Patel KK, Pye KL, Rodak J Jr, Veit KJ, Wood DL. 2001. Innovative approaches to educating medical students for practice in a changing health care environment: the National UME-21 Project. *Academic Medicine.* 76(6): 587-597.

Ramirez AJ, Graham J, Richards MA, Cull A, Gregory WM, Leaning MS, Snashall DC, Timothy AR. 1995. Burnout and psychiatric disorder among cancer clinicians. *British Journal of Cancer.* 71(6): 1263-1269.

Rao JK, Weinberger M, Kroenke K. 2000. Visit-specific expectations and patient-centered outcomes: a literature review. *Archives of Family Medicine.* 9(10): 1148-1155.

Rasmussen AF Jr, Marsh JT, Brill NQ. 1957. Increased susceptibility to herpes simplex in mice subjected to avoidance-learning stress or restraint. *Proceedings of the Society for Experimental Biology and Medicine.* 96(1): 183-189.

Reid SA, Glasser M. 1997. Primary care physicians' recognition of and attitudes toward domestic violence. *Academic Medicine.* 72(1): 51-53.

Reuben DB. 1983. Psychologic effects of residency. *Southern Medical Journal.* 76(3): 380-383.

Ritchie MA. 2001. Sources of emotional support for adolescents with cancer. *Journal of Pediatric Oncology Nursing.* 18(3):105-110.

Robins LS, White CB, Fantone JC. 2000. The difficulty of sustaining curricular reforms: a study of "drift" at one school. *Academic Medicine.* 75(8): 801-805.

Rosal MC, Ockene IS, Ockene JK, Barrett SV, Ma Y, Hebert JR. 1997. A longitudinal study of students' depression at one medical school. *Academic Medicine.* 72(6): 542-546.

Roter D, Kinmonth AL. 2002. What is the evidence that increasing participation of individuals in self-management improves the processes and outcomes of care? In: Williams R, Kinmonth A, Wareham M, Herman W, Eds. *The Evidence Base for Diabetes Care.* Chichester, England: John Wiley and Sons.

Roter DL, Hall JA, Kern DE, Barker LR, Cole KA, Roca RP. 1995. Improving physicians' interviewing skills and reducing patients' emotional distress. A randomized clinical trial. *Archives of Internal Medicine.* 155(17): 1877-1884.

Roter DL, Stewart M, Putnam SM, Lipkin M Jr, Stiles W, Inui TS. 1997. Communication patterns of primary care physicians. *Journal of the American Medical Association.* 277(4): 350-356.

Rothchild E. 1994. Family dynamics in end-of-life treatment decisions. *General Hospital Psychiatry.* 16(4): 251-258.

Ruschitzka F, Meier PJ, Turina M, Luscher TF, Noll G. 2000. Acute heart transplant rejection due to St John's wort. *Lancet.* 355(9203): 548-549.

Sacco RL, Elkind M, Boden-Albala B, Lin IF, Kargman DE, Hauser WA, Shea S, Paik MC. 1999. The protective effect of moderate alcohol consumption on ischemic stroke. *Journal of the American Medical Association.* 281(1): 53-60.

Sachdeva AK. 2000. Faculty development and support needed to integrate the learning of prevention in the curricula of medical schools. *Academic Medicine.* 75(7): 35S-42S.

Safran DG, Taira DA, Rogers WH, Kosinski M, Ware JE, Tarlov AR. 1998. Linking primary care performance to outcomes of care. *Journal of Family Practice*. 47(3): 213-220.

Satterfield JM, Mitteness LS, Tervalon M, Adler N. 2004. Integrating the social and behavioral sciences in an undergraduate medical curriculum: the UCSF essential core. *Academic Medicine*. 79(1): 6-15.

Schiffrin A. 2001. Psychosocial issues in pediatric diabetes. *Current Diabetes Reports*. 1(1): 33-40.

Schmidt HG, Norman GR, Boshuizen HP. 1990. A cognitive perspective on medical expertise: theory and implication. *Academic Medicine*. 65(10): 611-621.

Schnall PL, Landsbergis PA, Baker D. 1994. Job strain and cardiovascular disease. *Annual Review of Public Health*. 15: 381-411.

Schroeder SA, Zones JS, Showstack JA. 1989. Academic medicine as a public trust. *Journal of the American Medical Association*. 262(6): 803-812.

Schwenk TL, Romano SE. 1992. Managing the difficult physician-patient relationship. *American Family Physician*. 46(5): 1503-1509.

Shanafelt TD, Bradley KA, Wipf JE, Back AL. 2002. Burnout and self-reported patient care in an internal medicine residency program. *Annals of Internal Medicine*. 136(5): 358-367.

Shanafelt TD, Sloan JA, Habermann TM. 2003. The well-being of physicians. *American Journal of Medicine*. 114(6): 513-519.

Shapiro SL, Schwartz GE, Bonner G. 1998. Effects of mindfulness-based stress reduction on medical and premedical students. *Journal of Behavioral Medicine*. 21(6): 581-599.

Sheehan DV, Ballenger J, Jacobsen G. 1980. Treatment of endogenous anxiety with phobic, hysterical, and hypochondriacal symptoms. *Archives of General Psychiatry*. 37(1): 51-59.

Sholevar GP, Perkel R. 1990. Family systems intervention and physical illness. *General Hospital Psychiatry*. 12(6): 363-372.

Silver HK, Glicken AD. 1990. Medical student abuse: incidence, severity, and significance. *Journal of the American Medical Association*. 263(4): 527-532.

Singh BS. 1998. Managing somatoform disorders. *Medical Journal of Australia*. 168(11): 572-577.

Skochelak S, Barley G, Fogarty J. 2001. What did we learn about leadership in medical education? Effecting institutional change through the interdisciplinay generalist curriculum project. *Academic Medicine*. 76(4): 86-90.

Smith GR. 1992. The epidemiology and treatment of depression when it coexists with somatoform disorders, somatization, or pain. *General Hospital Psychiatry*. 14(4): 265-272.

Smith JW, Denny WF, Witzke DB. 1986. Emotional impairment in internal medicine house staff: results of a national survey. *Journal of the American Medical Association*. 255(9): 1155-1158.

Smith RC. 1996. *The Patient's Story*. Boston: Little, Brown, and Co.

Sobel DS. 2000. The cost-effectiveness of mind-body medicine interventions. *Progress in Brain Research*. 122: 393-412.

Spiro HM. 1993. What is empathy and can it be taught? In: Sprio HM, Curnen MGM, Peschel E, James DS, Eds. *Empathy and the Practice of Medicine*. New Haven, CT: Yale University Press.

Stalburg CM, Stein TA. 2002. An interdisciplinary course in women's health integrating basic and clinical sciences: clinical anatomy and women's health. *American Journal of Obstetrics and Gynecology*. 187(3 Suppl): S49-S52.

Steele DJ, Susman JL. 1998. Integrated clinical experience: University of Nebraska Medical Center. *Academic Medicine*. 73(1): 41-47.

Stein HF. 1985. *The Psychodynamics of Medical Practice*. Berkley, CA: University of California Press.

Steinert Y, Nasmith L, McLeod PJ, Conochie L. 2003. A teaching scholars program to develop leaders in medical education. *Academic Medicine*. 78(2): 142-149.

Steinmetz D, Tabenkin H. 2001. The "difficult patient" as perceived by family physicians. *Family Practice*. 18(5): 495-500.

Stewart M, Brown JB, Weston WW, McWhinney IR, McWilliam CL, Freeman TR. 1995. *Patient Centered Medicine*. Thousand Oaks, CA: Sage.

Stewart M, Brown JB, Boon H, Galajda J, Meredith L, Sangster M. 1999. Evidence on patient-doctor communication. *Cancer Prevention and Control*. 3(1): 25-30.

Stine C, Kohrs FP, Little DN, Kaprielian V, Gatipon BB, Haq C. 2000. Integrating prevention education into the medical school curriculum: the role of departments of family medicine. *Academic Medicine*. 75(7 Suppl): S55-S59.

Stoeckle JD, Billings JA. 1987. A history of history-taking: the medical interview. *Journal of General Internal Medicine*. 2(2): 119-127.

Straus R. 1996. A Philosophy of Medical Education for the University of Kentucky College of Medicine. In: *A Medical School Is Born*. Kuttawa, KY: McClanahan Publishing.

Studdert DM, Bhattacharya J, Schoenbaum M, Warren B, Escarce JJ. 2002. Personal choices of health plans by managed care experts. *Medical Care*. 40(5): 375-386.

Sugarman J, Burk L. 1998. Physicians' ethical obligations regarding alternative medicine. *Journal of the American Medical Association*. 280(18): 1623-1625.

Swanson DB, Case SM, Melnick DE, Volle RL. 1992. Impact of the USMLE step 1 on teaching and learning of the basic biomedical sciences. United States Medical Licensing Examination. *Academic Medicine*. 67(9): 553-556.

Tang TS, Fantone JC, Bozynski MEA, Adams BS. 2002. Implementation and evaluation of an undergraduate sociocultural medicine program. *Academic Medicine*. 77(6): 578-585.

Taylor JS. 2003a. Confronting "culture" in medicine's "culture of no culture". *Academic Medicine*. 78(6): 555-559.

Taylor JS. 2003b. The story catches you and you fall down: tragedy, ethnography, and "cultural competence". *Medical Anthropology Quarterly*. 17(2): 159-181.

Thibault GE, Neill JM, Lowenstein DH. 2003. The Academy at Harvard Medical School: nurturing teaching and stimulating innovation. *Academic Medicine*. 78(7): 673-81.

Thompson RS, Rivara FP, Thompson DC, Barlow WE, Sugg NK, Maiuro RD, Rubanowice DM. 2000. Identification and management of domestic violence: a randomized trial. *American Journal of Preventive Medicine*. 19(4): 253-263.

Todd KH, Samaroo N, Hoffman JR. 1993. Ethnicity as a risk factor for inadequate emergency department analgesia. *Journal of the American Medical Association*. 269(12): 1537-1539.

Tosteson DGH. 1994. Lessons for the future. In: Tosteson D, Adelstein S, Carver S, Eds. *New Pathways to Medical Education: Learning to Learn at Harvard Medical School*. Cambridge, MA: Harvard University Press.

Tsigos C, Chrousos GP. 2002. Hypothalamic-pituitary-adrenal axis, neuroendocrine factors and stress. *Journal of Psychosomatic Research*. 53(4): 865-871.

Turk DC, Okifuji A. 2002. Psychological factors in chronic pain: evolution and revolution. *Journal of Consulting and Clinical Psychology*. 70(3): 678-690.

UCSF (University of California, San Fransisco). 2003. *UCSF School of Medicine*. [Online] Available: http://medschool.ucsf.edu/ [accessed November 2003].

University of Rochester. 2002. *Overview of the Four-Year Curriculum*. Rochester, NY: University of Rochester School of Medicine and Dentistry.

University of Wisconsin. 2003. *Cardiovascular Medicine Handbook*. [Online] Available: http://app.medicine.wisc.edu/cardiobook/displayintro.cfm?page=1 [accessed October 2003].

U.S. Bureau of the Census. 1996. *Current Population Reports*. Population Projections of the United States by Age, Sex, Race, and Hispanic Origin: 1995 to 2050. Washington, DC: U.S. Department of Commerce, Bureau of the Census.

U.S. DHHS (U.S. Department of Health and Human Services). 1996. *Physical Activity and Health: A Report of the U.S. Surgeon General*. Atlanta, GA: Centers for Disease Control and Prevention.

U.S. DHHS. 1999. *Mental Health: A Report of the Surgeon General.* Rockville, MD: U.S. Department of Health and Human Services, Substance Abuse and Mental Health Services Administration, Center for Mental Health Services, National Institutes of Health, National Institute of Mental Health.

U.S. DHHS. 2000a. *Healthy People 2010: Understanding and Improving Health.* Washington, DC: U.S. Government Printing Office.

U.S. DHHS. 2000b. *Reducing Tobacco Use: A Report of the Surgeon General.* Office on Smoking and Health. Atlanta, GA: U.S. Department of Health and Human Services, Centers for Disease Control and Prevention.

U.S. DHHS. 2001. *The Surgeon General's Call to Action to Prevent and Decrease Overweight and Obesity.* Rockville, MD: Office of the Surgeon General, U.S. Department of Health and Human Services, Public Health Service.

Valmadrid CT, Klein R, Moss SE, Klein BE, Cruickshanks KJ. 1999. Alcohol intake and the risk of coronary heart disease mortality in persons with older-onset diabetes mellitus. *Journal of the American Medical Association.* 282(3): 239-246.

van Jaarsveld CH, Sanderman R, Miedema I, Ranchor AV, Kempen GI. 2001. Changes in health-related quality of life in older patients with acute myocardial infarction or congestive heart failure: a prospective study. *Journal of the American Geriatrics Society.* 49(8): 1052-1058.

van Ryn M, Burke J. 2000. The effect of patient race and socio-economic status on physicians' perceptions of patients. *Social Science and Medicine.* 50(6): 813-828.

Veloski JJ, Rabinowitz HK, Robeson MR, Young PR. 1999. Patients don't present with five choices: an alternative to multiple-choice tests in assessing physicians' competence. *Academic Medicine.* 74(5): 539-546.

Vitaliano PP, Maiuro RD, Russo J, Mitchell ES, Carr JE, Van Citters RL. 1988. A biopsychosocial model of medical student distress. *Journal of Behavioral Medicine.* 11(4): 311-331.

Vitaliano PP, Maiuro RD, Russo J, Mitchell ES. 1989. Medical student distress: a longitudinal study. *Journal of Nervous and Mental Disease.* 177(2): 70-76.

Von Korff M, Gruman J, Schaefer J, Curry SJ, Wagner EH. 1997. Collaborative management of chronic illness. *Annals of Internal Medicine.* 127(12): 1097-1102.

Wadden TA, Berkowitz RI, Vogt RA, Steen SN, Stunkard AJ, Foster GD. 1997. Lifestyle modification in the pharmacologic treatment of obesity: a pilot investigation of a potential primary care approach. *Obesity Research.* 5(3): 218-226.

Wagner EH, Austin BT, Von Korff M. 1996. Improving outcomes in chronic illness. *Managed Care Quarterly.* 4(2): 12-25.

Wagner EH, Glasgow RE, Davis C, Bonomi AE, Provost L, McCulloch D, Carver P, Sixta C. 2001. Quality improvement in chronic illness care: a collaborative approach. *Joint Commission Journal on Quality Improvement.* 27(2): 63-80.

Waldstein SR, Neumann SA, Drossman DA, Novack DH. 2001. Teaching psychosomatic (biopsychosocial) medicine in United States medical schools: survey findings. *Psychosomatic Medicine.* 63(3): 335-343.

Walker CE, Hedberg A, Clement PW, Wright L. 1981. *Clinical Procedures for Behavior Therapy.* Englewood Cliffs, NJ: Prentice-Hall.

Walker EA, Gelfand AN, Gelfand MD, Koss MP, Katon WJ. 1995. Medical and psychiatric symptoms in female gastroenterology clinic patients with histories of sexual victimization. *General Hospital Psychiatry.* 17(2): 85-92.

Walker EA, Katon WJ, Keegan D, Gardner G, Sullivan M. 1997. Predictors of physician frustration in the care of patients with rheumatological complaints. *General Hospital Psychiatry.* 19(5): 315-323.

Warde CM, Moonesinghe K, Allen W, Gelberg L. 1999. Marital and parental satisfaction of married physicians with children. *Journal of General Internal Medicine.* 14(3): 157-165.

Warshaw C. 1997. Intimate partner abuse: developing a framework for change in medical education. *Academic Medicine.* 72(1 Suppl): S26-S37.

Warshaw C, Alpert E. 1999. Integrating routine inquiry about domestic violence into daily practice. *Annals of Internal Medicine.* 131(8): 619-620.

Wartman S, Davis A, Wilson M, Kahn N, Sherwood R, Nowalk A. 2001. Curricular change: recommendations from a national perspective. *Academic Medicine.* 76(4 Suppl): S140-145.

Watson M, Haviland JS, Greer S, Davidson J, Bliss JM. 1999. Influence of psychological response on survival in breast cancer: a population-based cohort study. *Lancet.* 354(9187): 1331-1336.

Weiner EL, Swain GR, Wolf B, Gottlieb M. 2001. A qualitative study of physicians' own wellness-promotion practices. *Western Journal of Medicine.* 174(1): 19-23.

Weinstock M. 1997. Does prenatal stress impair coping and regulation of hypothalamic-pituitary-adrenal axis? *Neuroscience and Biobehavioral Reviews.* 21(1): 1-10.

Wennberg J, Gittelsohn A. 1973. Small area variations in health care delivery. *Science.* 182(117): 1102-1108.

Wennberg JE, Freeman JL, Culp WJ. 1987. Are hospital services rationed in New Haven or over-utilised in Boston? *Lancet.* 1(8543): 1185-1189.

Wetzel MS, Eisenberg DM, Kaptchuk TJ. 1998. Courses involving complementary and alternative medicine at US medical schools. *Journal of the American Medical Association.* 280(9): 784-787.

Wetzel MS, Kaptchuk TJ, Haramati A, Eisenberg DM. 2003. Complementary and alternative medical therapies: implications for medical education. *Annals of Internal Medicine.* 138(3): 191-196.

Whitehouse WG, Dinges DF, Orne EC, Keller SE, Bates BL, Bauer NK, Morahan P, Haupt BA, Carlin MM, Bloom PB, Zaugg L, Orne MT. 1996. Psychosocial and immune effects of self-hypnosis training for stress management throughout the first semester of medical school. *Psychosomatic Medicine.* 58(3): 249-263.

Whitlock EP, Orleans CT, Pender N, Allan J. 2002. Evaluating primary care behavioral counseling interventions: an evidence-based approach. *American Journal of Preventive Medicine.* 22(4): 267-284.

Whooley MA, Simon GE. 2000. Managing depression in medical outpatients. *New England Journal of Medicine.* 343(26): 1942-1950.

Wilkerson L, Irby DM. 1998. Strategies for improving teaching practices: a comprehensive approach to faculty development. *Academic Medicine.* 73(4): 387-396.

Wilkes MS, Usatine R, Slavin S, Hoffman JR. 1998. Doctoring: University of California, Los Angeles. *Academic Medicine.* 73(1): 32-40.

Williams GC, Freedman ZR, Deci EL. 1998. Supporting autonomy to motivate patients with diabetes for glucose control. *Diabetes Care.* 21(10): 1644-1651.

Williams JK, Vita JA, Manuck SB, Selwyn AP, Kaplan JR. 1991. Psychosocial factors impair vascular responses of coronary arteries. *Circulation.* 84(5): 2146-2153.

Williamson P, Beitman BD, Katon W. 1981. Beliefs that foster physician avoidance of psychosocial aspects of health care. *Journal of Family Practice.* 13(7): 999-1003.

Williamson PR. 1992. Support groups: an important aspect of physician education. *Journal of General Internal Medicine.* 6: 179-180.

Wilson PW, D'Agostino RB, Levy D, Belanger AM, Silbershatz H, Kannel WB. 1998. Prediction of coronary heart disease using risk factor categories. *Circulation.* 97(18): 1837-1847.

Wojcik BE, Spinks MK, Optenberg SA. 1998. Breast carcinoma survival analysis for African American and white women in an equal-access health care system. *Cancer.* 82(7): 1310-1318.

Yedidia MJ, Gillespie CC, Kachur E, Schwartz MD, Ockene J, Chepaitis AE, Snyder CW, Lazare A, Lipkin M Jr. 2003. Effect of communications training on medical student performance. *Journal of the American Medical Association.* 290(9): 1157-1165.

A

Methods

This appendix describes the methods used by the committee to collect information for its review, assessment, and consideration. Four types of data collection were undertaken: a literature review, invited presentations, a survey of selected medical schools, and a modified Delphi process for prioritizing topics (see Chapter 3). Each activity is described below.

LITERATURE REVIEW

The committee's initial literature search (Figure A-1) concentrated on journals found in the MEDLINE database. A second, expanded literature search (Figure A-2) included multiple databases. As noted throughout this report, these searches yielded a relatively small number of articles specific to the inclusion of the behavioral and social sciences in medical education. Broad search terms were used to cast as wide a net as possible. The articles obtained by the search terms were reviewed for their relevance to the committee's charge. To be viewed as relevant for this report, an article had to be in English and meet one of the following criteria: (1) describe or review medical school curriculum content identified as relevant to the behavioral and social sciences; (2) describe or review medical school curricula or curriculum change; or (3) include a discussion of undergraduate medical school education.

Systematic reviews or descriptions of behavioral and social science content in undergraduate medical school curricula were not found. Articles describing the rationale or goals of a behavioral and social science program, including examples of course content, were obtained. However, these articles did not provide enough information to allow a review of the approaches that have been or are successful

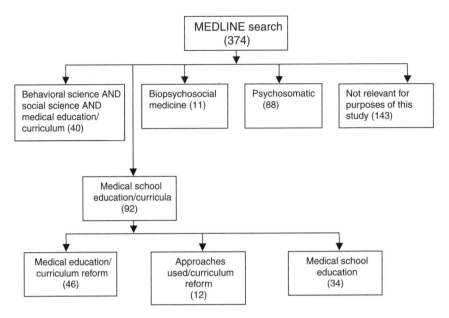

FIGURE A-1 MEDLINE search results. The numbers in parentheses indicate the number of articles found in each category; some articles fall under more than one category. The search was limited by language (English), species (human), and year (1970–2003).

in teaching the behavioral and social sciences in medical school or an evaluation of the effectiveness of current programs. The majority of the articles describing or reviewing curriculum change were not specific to the behavioral and social sciences, but were deemed to address overarching principles and strategies applicable to these disciplines.

INVITED PRESENTATIONS

The committee held multiple open sessions at which invited speakers representing interested organizations, associations, and medical schools provided information. During the sessions, the committee was able to discuss the information presented and gain additional insight from different perspectives regarding the inclusion of the behavioral and social sciences in medical school curricula. A list of the associations, organizations, medical schools, and respective institutions represented by the invited speakers appears in Box A-1.

MEDICAL SCHOOL SURVEY

To obtain additional information on the current status of behavioral and social science content in medical school curricula, the committee surveyed a lim-

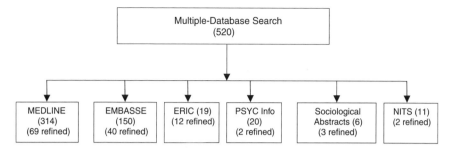

FIGURE A-2 Results of electronic multiple-database search. The numbers in parentheses indicate the number of articles found in each database. The second number in parentheses (refined) indicates the number of articles that remained after nonrelevant articles had been eliminated. The following search terms were used: Medical, Faculty, Education, Undergraduate, Behavioral Sciences, and Social Sciences. Articles with the following terms as a primary focus were eliminated from the search to create the refined results: Distance Education, Informatics, Forensic/Autopsy, Residency, Health Professions other than physician, Medical Subspecialties, Career Planning, Nuclear Medicine, Master of Business Administration, and Bioterrorism. The search was limited by language (English) and year (1995–2003).

ited number of medical schools using a two-step data collection method. Four schools were selected and surveyed based on initial information that indicated their behavioral and social science program could serve as an example of current approaches being used. The survey consisted of two parts: a brief questionnaire completed by an official of the medical school, followed by a telephone interview with that individual. The four schools surveyed were Ohio State University College of Medicine; University of California, San Francisco, School of Medicine; University of Rochester Medical Center; and University of North Carolina School of Medicine.

MODIFIED DELPHI PROCESS

The committee used a modified Delphi process to establish the priority topics delineated in Chapter 3. The initial step was to establish a list of all possible topics in the behavioral and social sciences that could be included in a curriculum for medical students (see Box A-2). The topics on this list varied in subject area, specificity of material, and level of relevance to undergraduate medical school education. Background materials that aided in establishing the original list encompassed (1) relevant, evidence-based articles and reports in the literature; (2) presentations to the committee by content experts and medical school representatives; (3) literature and other material from the Association of American Medical Colleges and the Liaison Committee on Medical Education; (4) considerations related to the health of the public, driven mainly by root causes of morbidity and

BOX A-1
List of Interested Associations, Organizations, and Medical Schools Represented by Invited Speakers

Association of American Medical Colleges
Association for the Behavioral Sciences and Medical Education
Brody School of Medicine, East Carolina University
Liaison Committee on Medical Education
National Board of Medical Examiners
Society of Behavioral Medicine
The Society of Teachers of Family Medicine
University of California, San Francisco
University of Rochester Medical Center

mortality; and (5) the gap between what is known and what is actually done in practice.

The committee's collective and individual experience in curriculum development and reform in the behavioral and social sciences largely directed the prioritization of the topics on the original list. The rating scale used to prioritize the topics ranged from 0 to 3, with 0 being the lowest score, and included "U" (for unknown) as an option for rating a topic if the level of priority was unknown or could not be determined by a committee member. Each topic was then assigned high, low, or medium priority based on its mean score and standard deviation.

Given the number of topics with large standard deviations, it was determined that a second round of ratings was needed to clarify the appropriate rating for each topic. For the second round of ratings, several decisions were made:

• Topics ranked as low or with a mean score equal to or less than 1 were removed from the list.
• Topics added by a committee member were placed as the first item in the appropriate category or subcategory.
• Committee members were given the opportunity to provide a rationale or clarification for their ratings.

The results of this second round provided additional clarification of topics, and the variance in standard deviations was reduced.

The next step in developing the list was to apply the following set of criteria:

• Is the content of this topic included in or overlapping with other topics on the list?

- Is undergraduate medical school the most appropriate level for this topic to be taught?
- Is the topic of limited value for general physician education?
- Is the topic part of a core behavioral or social science curriculum?

Based on a combination of the answers to the above questions, mean scores, standard deviations, and the expert opinion of the committee, topics were removed from the list and/or reassigned high, medium, or low priority. The committee reviewed a third ranked list and performed a final rating, this time using a 0 to 5 scale similar to the one discussed previously. This list was refined and finalized using the collective and individual expertise of the committee members in medical school curriculum development and reform in the behavioral and social sciences. The final list of topics is in Chapter 3, Table 3-1. In this list, the 11 items ranked top and the 9 items ranked high were combined into one high-priority group.

BOX A-2
Suggested Curriculum Content Organized by Five Domains

Biological Domain
Psychological Domain
Social Domain
Behavioral Domain
Economic Domain

1.0   Biological Domain

1.1   Genetic contributions to behavior
    1.1.1   Concepts in behavioral genetics
    1.1.2   Assessment of genetic contributions to personality and behavior
    1.1.3   Principles and strategies of genetic counseling

1.2   Mind–body interactions in health and disease
    1.2.1   Brain/behavior/central nervous system/autonomic nervous system
    1.2.2   Psychoendocrinology
    1.2.3   Psychoneuroimmunology
    1.2.4   Pathobiology
    1.2.5   Biological basis of illness behavior

1.3   Mind–body interactions in specific disease states
    1.3.1   Cardiovascular diseases
    1.3.2   Gastrointestinal diseases
    1.3.3   HIV/AIDS
    1.3.4   Neurological disorders, e.g. Parkinson's disease, frontal tumors, chronic pain
    1.3.5   Mood disorders
    1.3.6   Substance abuse
    1.3.7   Sleep disorders
    1.3.8   Eating disorders
    1.3.9   Psychosis

2.0   Psychological Domain

2.1   Psychological models of human behavior
    2.1.1   Cognitive psychology: thinking habits, core schemas (Beck), focus of control (Roter), cognitive dissonance (Festinger), "transtheoretical" psychology of change (Prochaska)
    2.1.2   Social psychology: roles and expectations, attributions, choice

2.1.3 Dynamic psychology: unconscious conflict, ego defenses

2.1.4 Social–cognitive models: self-efficacy, coping models (Bandura)

2.1.5 Systems theory: family dynamics, functions of the sick member

2.1.6 Humanistic psychology: empathy, warmth, genuineness (Rogers)

2.1.7 Personality development and personality types (Shapiro, *Diagnostic and Statistical Manual* [DSM]-IV)

2.1.8 Normal development: birth through old age

2.2 The psychology of patients

2.2.1 Expectations, biases, and assumptions about the nature of illness and the roles of doctor and patient: mind–body dualism

2.2.2 The psychology of health risk behaviors: food, tobacco, alcohol and substance abuse, risky sex, risky driving, risky sports behaviors

2.2.3 Normal illness psychology: fear and anxiety, vulnerability, appropriate dependency, humiliation, anger, sadness, and loss

2.2.4 Abnormal illness psychology: denial, pathological dependency, depression, somatization, hypochondriasis

2.2.5 The psychology of somatoform disorders (e.g., lower back pain, irritable bowel syndrome, chronic fatigue syndrome)

2.2.6 The psychology of chronic pain

2.2.7 Psychological issues in chronic diseases and disabilities

2.2.8 Psychopathology—DSM-IV disorders

2.3 The psychology of doctors

2.3.1 Expectations, biases, and assumptions about the nature of illness and the roles of doctor and patient: mind–body dualism

2.3.2 Knowledge availability: memory structures, pattern recognition

2.3.3 The processes of clinical reasoning: reflective and analytic versus gestalt and associative reasoning ("knee-jerk reactions"); hypothetical deductive reasoning, etc.

2.3.4 Shared decision making (clinician–clinician and clinician–patient)

Continued

BOX A-2 Continued

2.3.5 The interpretation of evidence
    2.3.5.1 Unwarranted variations in health care delivery
        (Wennberg)
2.3.6 Effects of informatics and other decision support systems
2.3.7 Effects of continuing medical education and recertification
    on clinical decision making
2.3.8 Dangers of stress and burnout: need for self-awareness,
    self-care

2.4 The psychology of doctor–patient relationships
    2.4.1 Doctor-centered: paternalistic, sole expert, etc.
    2.4.2 Patient-centered: activated patient, patient as expert
    2.4.3 Relationship-centered

3.0 Social Domain

3.1 Basic concepts
    3.1.1 Social stresses and supports as determinants of health
    3.1.2 The sick role as a social construct
    3.1.3 The professional role and ethics as social constructs
    3.1.4 Health care policies
    3.1.5 Clinical medicine and public health
    3.1.6 High-risk versus population-based approaches
    3.1.7 Community health
    3.1.8 Levels of organization in health care
    3.1.9 Occupational health
    3.1.10 Evaluating individual context (e.g., available
        tangible support); capacity for self-care, making
        medical decisions, and independent living

3.2 Multicultural medicine
    3.2.1 Cultural competence in diagnosis
    3.2.2 Cultural competence in patient management
    3.2.3 Cultural issues in patient–physician interactions
    3.2.4 Folk medicine, alternative medicine, and biomedical
        treatment

3.3 Social inequalities in health
    3.3.1 Social inequalities in health care
    3.3.2 Poverty/homelessness
    3.3.3 Rural/urban issues and culture

3.4 Gender issues in health care

3.5 Sexual orientation issues in health care

3.6 Domestic abuse, violence

3.7 Social constraints on physician behavior
    3.7.1 Health maintenance organization requirements
    3.7.2 Insurance carriers
    3.7.3 Legal risk and malpractice insurance
    3.7.4 Medical jurisprudence
    3.7.5 Confidentiality issues

3.8 Social influences on physician behavior
    3.8.1 Social accountability and responsibility
    3.8.2 Professional norms for referrals, case management, and follow-up
    3.8.3 Culture of biomedicine, including cultures of training environments
    3.8.4 Medical humanities

3.9 Social change
    3.9.1 Communication behavior change (McGuire)
    3.9.2 Diffusion of innovation (Rogers)
    3.9.3 Social marketing
    3.9.4 Social change theories
    3.9.5 Economic incentive theories
    3.9.6 Public policy and advocacy

3.10 Medical practice organization to ensure optimal care delivery

3.11 Effective use of community resources to enhance care

4.0 Behavioral Domain

4.1 Principles of behavior management: accurate assessment and goal setting, contingent reinforcement and stimulus conditioning

4.2 Maladaptive behavior patterns of patients
    4.2.1 Health risk behaviors: abuse of alcohol, nicotine, illegal drugs, legal drugs, unhealthy foods: over- and undereating; risk taking in sexual activities, sports, and driving: deliberate self-harm and self-mutilation; fictitious illness (Munchausen syndrome and malingering)

Continued

BOX A-2 Continued

4.2.2 Maladaptive help-seeking behaviors: high-frequency attendance; nonadherence, including appointment nonattendance; demanding or critical behavior; flattering or seductive behavior; dependent behavior

4.3 Maladaptive behavior patterns of doctors

4.3.1 Poor communication skills: Inattentive listening or failure to check and clarify diagnostic data, failure to elicit psychosocial data, failure to demonstrate empathy and respect or to promote partnership, failure to explore patient's views about diagnosis and treatment, failure to give adequate explanations of diagnosis and treatment

4.3.2 Lapses in professional role behavior: poor timekeeping, excess formality or informality, failure to maintain professional boundaries in relating to patients, failure to maintain updated knowledge and skills, inadequate attention to psychosocial/behavioral and somatoform problems

4.4 Communication skills for doctors

4.4.1 Basic concepts: process versus content, structure versus function, skills versus attitudes continued

4.4.2 Skills for building a therapeutic relationship, e.g., empathy, respect, support

4.4.3 Skills for eliciting data for a five-domain assessment, e.g., open questions, active listening, checking and clarifying

4.4.4 Skills for educating, advising, and promoting behavior change: e.g., creating links with patient's knowledge and experience

4.4.5 Advanced communication competencies; giving bad news; dealing with patients' and families' anger, diagnosing and counseling for obesity, alcoholism, smoking, substance abuse, risky sexual behaviors, domestic abuse, depression, etc.

5.0 Economic Domain

5.1 Overview of the U.S. health care system

5.1.1 Public insurance

5.1.2 Employer provision of health insurance

5.1.3 Insurance models

5.1.4 Hospital markets

5.2 Patient behavior
   5.2.1 Risk
   5.2.2 Health production
   5.2.3 Problems of asymmetric information between doctor and patient

5.3 Health insurance
   5.3.1 Demand for health insurance
   5.3.2 Welfare loss or excess insurance (moral hazard)
   5.3.3 Employer-provided health insurance and job lock

5.4 Provider behavior
   5.4.1 Physician-induced demand
   5.4.2 Hospital competition

5.5 Trade-offs among efficiency, equity, and selection
   5.5.1 Prospective payment
   5.5.2 Fee-for-service payment
   5.5.3 Risk selection in health plans

5.6 Quantitative methods in health economics
   5.6.1 Prediction versus causation in health economics
   5.6.2 Randomized controlled trials and the causation problem
   5.6.3 Outcomes analyses (natural experiments)

5.7 Health policy
   5.7.1 The problem of the uninsured and public insurance crowd-out effects
   5.7.2 Mandated health insurance benefits and employment effects
   5.7.3 Hospital competition and medical arms race
   5.7.4 Racial and educational disparities in health care
   5.7.5 Are medical care prices really rising?
   5.7.6 Quality report cards and consumer choice
   5.7.7 Prescription drug benefits and costs
   5.7.8 Direct-to-consumer advertising of pharmaceuticals
   5.7.9 Community rating and adverse selection
   5.7.10 Price controls in insurance markets

QUESTIONNAIRE SENT TO MEDICAL SCHOOLS

1.   At your school, the primary strategy for teaching behavioral and social science material is: primarily: (Please circle the appropriate letter)
  a.   Integrated as a content theme across several course in the curricula. Taught as a content theme in more than two courses in the curricula
  b.   Concentrated in a few courses.

2.   Please complete the chart below.

Please indicate if this information is taught by checking yes or no	YES	NO	Title of course(s) that includes information	Department(s) responsible for teaching behavioral and social science content	Circle Year Taught	Teaching method* (circle all that apply)
Communication Skills	❏	❏			1 2 3 4	PBL SG L U O
Community Health	❏	❏			1 2 3 4	PBL SG L U O
Cultural Diversity	❏	❏			1 2 3 4	PBL SG L U O
End of Life Care	❏	❏			1 2 3 4	PBL SG L U O
Epidemiology	❏	❏			1 2 3 4	PBL SG L U O
Family/Domestic Violence	❏	❏			1 2 3 4	PBL SG L U O

QUESTIONNAIRE SENT TO MEDICAL SCHOOLS (Continued)

Please indicate if this information is taught by checking yes or no	YES	NO	Title of course(s) that includes information	Department(s) responsible for teaching behavioral and social science content	Circle Year Taught	Teaching method* (circle all that apply)
Health Care Quality Improvement	❑	❑			1 2 3 4	PBL SG L U O
Health Care Systems	❑	❑			1 2 3 4	PBL SG L U O
Health Literacy	❑	❑			1 2 3 4	PBL SG L U O
Human Development/ Life Cycle	❑	❑			1 2 3 4	PBL SG L U O
Medical Social Economics	❑	❑			1 2 3 4	PBL SG L U O
Pain Management	❑	❑			1 2 3 4	PBL SG L U O
Palliative Care	❑	❑			1 2 3 4	PBL SG L U O

Continued

QUESTIONNAIRE SENT TO MEDICAL SCHOOLS (Continued)

Please indicate if this information is taught by checking yes or no	YES	NO	Title of course(s) that includes information	Department(s) responsible for teaching behavioral and social science content	Circle Year Taught	Teaching method* (circle all that apply)
Patient Health Education	❑	❑			1 2 3 4	PBL SG L U O
Population based Medicine	❑	❑			1 2 3 4	PBL SG L U O
Prevention and Health Maintenance	❑	❑			1 2 3 4	PBL SG L U O
Substance Abuse	❑	❑			1 2 3 4	PBL SG L U O

*L = lecture, PBL = problem based learning, SG = small-group, U = unknown, O = other (describe).

1. Does your school provide formal faculty development in behavioral and social science content for participation in these courses? (Circle the appropriate letter.)
    a. Yes
    b. No

2. Is there a faculty or staff position that is principally responsible for faculty development? (Circle the appropriate letter.)
    a. Yes, please provide the position title _____
    b. No

3. What activities are part of your formal faculty development program? (Circle all that apply.)
    a. Small group discussions
    b. Demonstrating/teaching techniques of problem-based learning
    c. Examples of incorporating behavioral and social science into clinical exam

d. Career development awards for behavioral and social science
e. Formal didactic sessions teaching faculty behavioral and social science material
f. Other _____
g. None

4. What rationale, if any, was stated as the primary reason for including this behavioral and social sciences content in the curriculum? (Circle all that apply.)

a, Meets licensing or accreditation requirement(s)
b. Better prepare medical students to care for patients
c. Communicates belief in multilevel approach to disease
d. Supports mission of the school
e. Meets societal expectations
f. Other _____
g. No formal rationale explicitly stated

5. There are several other topics of relevance to your behavioral/social science curriculum we would like to explore with a key, knowledgeable person in a telephone appointment of 15-20 minutes' length. Whom should we contact for this appointment and conversation?

Name _____
Telephone number _____
E-mail address _____

THANK YOU

B

Committee and Staff Biographies

Neal A. Vanselow, M.D., *Chair*, is Professor Emeritus of Medicine at Tulane University Health Sciences Center. He also holds appointments as Professor Emeritus of Health Systems Management in the Tulane School of Public Health and Tropical Medicine and as an Adjunct Professor in the School of Health Administration and Policy at Arizona State University. He is a former Chancellor of Tulane University Medical Center and past chairman of the Council on Graduate Medical Education of the U.S. Department of Health and Human Services. He has also served as chairman of the Board of Directors, Association of Academic Health Centers, and as a Senior Scholar in Residence at the Institute of Medicine. He has been a member of the Pew Health Professions Commission and the University of California Commission on the Future of Medical Education. Dr. Vanselow's areas of expertise include medical center administration, allergy/immunology, and health professions education. His research interests have focused on the health care workforce, undergraduate and graduate medical education, and regulation of the health professions. He chaired the Institute of Medicine's Committee on the Future of Primary Care and served as cochair of the Institute of Medicine's Committee on the U.S. Physician Supply. He has also chaired the Continuing Evaluation Panel of the American International Health Alliance. Dr. Vanselow is a member of the Board of Trustees of Meharry Medical College and a member of the Institute of Medicine.

Robert Daugherty Jr., M.D., Ph.D., is Dean (emeritus) of the University of South Florida College of Medicine and Vice President of the Health Sciences Center. His areas of expertise include medical education, internal medicine, and physiology. His former positions include Dean and Professor of Medicine at the

University of Nevada School of Medicine; Associate Dean and Director of Continuing Medical Education at Indiana University School of Medicine; Dean and Assistant to the President at the College of Human Medicine, University of Wyoming; and acting Associate Dean and Director of the Offices of Curriculum Implementation and Interdepartmental Curriculum, College of Human Medicine, Michigan State University. Dr. Daugherty is a member of the American Federation for Clinical Research, the American Medical Association, and the Central Society for Clinical Research. He has participated extensively in national medical education activities, including serving on the National Board of Medical Examiners and the Accreditation Council for Graduate Medical Education. He has also chaired the Liaison Committee on Medical Education and the Council of Deans of the Association of American Medical Colleges.

Peggye Dilworth-Anderson, Ph.D., is Professor of Health Policy and Administration at the School of Public Health and Director of the Center for Aging and Diversity at the University of North Carolina at Chapel Hill. Her areas of expertise include minority aging, caregiving to cognitively and physically dependent elders, and culture and family development. Dr. Dilworth-Anderson is currently serving on the Board of Directors of the Alzheimer's Association. She also serves on the editorial boards of several major journals in aging and in family studies. She is the recipient of a number of awards and honors for her work, and has numerous articles published and in press. She is a member of the American Sociological Association, the Gerontological Society of America, the National Council on Family Relations, and the American Public Health Association.

Karen Emmons, Ph.D., is Professor of Society, Human Development, and Health at the Harvard School of Public Health and a faculty member in the Center for Community-Based Research (CCBR) at the Dana-Farber Cancer Institute (DFCI). She is also Director of Tobacco Control at DFCI and Deputy Director of CCBR. Her expertise and major research interests include community-based approaches to cancer prevention and control; cancer disparities; motivation for health behavior change; health communication; cancer screening; tobacco control and smoking cessation; environmental tobacco smoke exposure; and behavior change interventions for other behavioral risk factors, including diet and exercise. Her teaching interests include psychosocial theories of health behavior and health and cancer communication. She is the author of numerous published peer-reviewed articles. She is a Member of the Academy of Behavioral Medicine Researchers and the Society of Behavioral Medicine.

Eugene K. Emory, Ph.D., is a clinical neuropsychologist and Professor in the Department of Psychology and the Department of Psychiatry and Behavioral Sciences at Emory University. He is also Director of Clinical Training in the University's Ph.D. program in clinical psychology. Dr. Emory is Director of the

Center for Prenatal Assessment and Human Development at Emory. His research in developmental and cognitive neuroscience focuses on prenatal brain–behavior relationships, incorporating both micro- and macrolevel analyses. His current research activities are devoted to computational models of prenatal brain, behavior, and cognition in humans and how these topics relate to normal development, mental health, and maternal psychopathology. Dr. Emory's previous work includes studies of fetal and infant neurobehavioral development and reproductive stress. He has served on a number of Institute of Medicine and National Research Council committees and is currently a member of the Board on Behavioral, Cognitive, and Sensory Sciences of the National Academy of Sciences.

Dana P. Goldman, Ph.D., holds the RAND Chair in Health Economics and is Director of RAND's Health Economics program. He is also an Adjunct Associate Professor in the David Geffen School of Medicine and School of Public Health at the University of California, Los Angeles. Dr. Goldman's research interests combine applied economics with health care delivery, with a focus on the economics of chronic illness. He was the recipient of the 2002 Alice S. Hersh New Investigator Award, which recognizes the contribution of scholars to the field of health services research. He also received the National Institute for Health Care Management Research and Educational Foundation award for excellence in health policy. Dr. Goldman is a Research Associate with the National Bureau of Economic Research and Director of the UCLA/RAND Postdoctoral Health Services Research Training Program.

Tana A. Grady-Weliky, M.D., is Senior Associate Dean for Medical Education and Associate Professor of Psychiatry and Obstetrics/Gynecology at the University of Rochester School of Medicine and Dentistry. Her expertise and research interests include personal and professional development of physicians across the medical education continuum (medical student to physician in practice), psychiatry residency education, psychopharmacology, and premenstrual dysphoria evaluation and treatment. Dr. Grady-Weliky previously taught at Howard, Georgetown, Duke, and Harvard Medical Schools. A number of her articles have been published in peer-reviewed journals. She is a member of the American Psychiatric Association, American Medical Association, Association of Women Psychiatrists, American College of Psychiatrists, Society for Executive Leadership in Academic Medicine, Society for Biological Psychiatry, American Medical Women's Association, and North American Society of Psychosomatic Obstetrics and Gynecology.

Thomas S. Inui, M.D., is President and CEO of the Regenstrief Institute for Health Care, Sam Regenstrief Professor of Health Services Research, and Associate Dean for Health Care Research at Indiana University School of Medicine. A primary care physician, educator, and researcher, he previously held positions as

Head of General Internal Medicine at the University of Washington School of Medicine and as Paul C. Cabot Professor and founding chair of the Department of Ambulatory Care and Prevention at Harvard Medical School. Dr. Inui's special emphases in teaching and research include physician–patient communication, health promotion and disease prevention, the social context of medicine, and medical humanities. His honors include elected membership in Phi Beta Kappa, Alpha Omega Alpha, and the Johns Hopkins University Society of Scholars; a U.S. Public Health Service Medal of Commendation; service as a member of the Council and President of the Society of General Internal Medicine; the Robert Glaser Award (for generalism); and election to the Institute of Medicine (and subsequently the Institute of Medicine Council).

David M. Irby, Ph.D., is Professor of Medicine, Vice Dean for Education, and Director of the Office of Medical Education at the University of California, San Francisco, School of Medicine. His areas of expertise include research on clinical teaching in medicine, faculty development, curriculum reform, and innovations in medical education. Dr. Irby was previously on the faculty at the University of Washington, where he directed the Center for Medical Education Research in the Department of Medical Education. For his research on clinical teaching and his leadership in medical education, he was awarded the Distinguished Scholar Award by the American Educational Research Association, the John P. Hubbard Award by the National Board of Medical Examiners, and the Daniel C. Tosteson Award for Leadership in Medical Education by the Carl J. Shapiro Institute for Education and Research at Beth Israel Deaconess Medical Center and Harvard Medical School. Dr. Irby is also noted for his publications and presentations on faculty development.

Dennis Novack, M.D., F.A.C.P., is Professor of Medicine and Associate Dean of Medical Education at Drexel University College of Medicine. His work has focused on clinical skills teaching and assessment, evaluation of the effectiveness of a variety of innovative educational programs, teaching and research in physician–patient communication, the influence of physician personal awareness and growth on well-being and clinical competence, psychosocial aspects of care, and medical ethics. He is Past President of the American Psychosomatic Society and Editor Emeritus of *Medical Encounter,* newsletter of the American Academy on Physician and Patient (AAPP). He and his colleagues in the AAPP are currently creating a comprehensive web resource on physician–patient communication, supported by the Arthur Vining Davis Foundation. Dr. Novack has published numerous articles, many of which are used in medical school courses throughout the world.

Neil Schneiderman, Ph.D., is James L. Knight Professor of Health Psychology, Medicine, Psychiatry and Behavioral Sciences, and Biomedical Engineering at the University of Miami. He is also Director of the university-wide Behavioral Medicine Research Center. His areas of expertise include biobehavioral aspects of cardiovascular disease, stress–endocrine–immune interactions, central nervous system control of circulation, AIDS, and noninvasive cardiovascular instrumentation. Dr. Schneiderman is Program Director for projects and research training grants for the National Institutes of Health (NIH). He has served as editor of two peer-reviewed scientific journals. He is a fellow of the Academy of Behavioral Medicine Research and American College of Clinical Pharmacology and former president of the International Society of Behavioral Medicine and the Academy of Behavioral Medicine Research. He has served as advisor to numerous national and international organizations, including NIH. Dr. Schneiderman is the recipient of distinguished scientific awards from the Society of Behavioral Medicine and the American Psychological Association.

Howard F. Stein, Ph.D., a medical and psychoanalytic anthropologist, has taught in the Department of Family and Preventive Medicine at the University of Oklahoma Health Sciences Center for 26 years. He is also director of the behavioral science curriculum at the rural Family Medicine residency program in Enid, Oklahoma. His expertise and research interests include the psychology of physician–patient–family relationships; ethnicity and health; rural medicine; trauma, loss, and grief; and occupational medicine. Dr. Stein was the recipient in 1998 of the Society of Teachers of Family Medicine Recognition Award for more than two decades of contributions to and leadership in the discipline of family medicine. He has authored and coauthored more than 200 articles and chapters and 24 books. He is past President of the High Plains Society for Applied Anthropology.

Institute of Medicine Staff

Andrew Pope, Ph.D., is director of the Board on Health Sciences Policy and the Board on Neuroscience and Behavioral Health at the Institute of Medicine. With a Ph.D. in physiology and biochemistry, his primary interests focus on environmental and occupational influences on human health. Dr. Pope's previous research activities focused on the neuroendocrine and reproductive effects of various environmental substances in food-producing animals. During his tenure at the National Academies and since 1989 at the Institute of Medicine, Dr. Pope has directed numerous studies; topics include injury control, disability prevention, biologic markers, neurotoxicology, indoor allergens, and the enhancement of environmental and occupational health content in medical and nursing school curricula. Most recently, Dr. Pope directed studies on NIH priority-setting processes, organ procurement and transplantation policy, and the role of science and technology in countering terrorism.

Lauren Honess-Morreale, M.P.H., was formerly study director for this study. Previously, she managed community-based research programs at the University of Texas School of Public Health, the M.D. Anderson Cancer Center, and the University of North Carolina at Chapel Hill. Her primary area of expertise is the application of behavior change and communication theories to the design and development of community-based programs. She has successfully managed large-scale multistate screening and health promotion programs. She earned her masters degree in public health at the Department of Health Behavior and Health Education at the University of North Carolina at Chapel Hill.

Patricia A. Cuff, M.S., R.D., M.P.H., succeeded Ms. Honess-Morreale as study director for this study. She joined the Institute of Medicine staff in April 2001 to work with the Board on Global Health on the report, *Microbial Threats to Health: Emergence, Detection, and Response.* Prior to that, Patricia worked extensively in the field of HIV–nutrition as a counselor, researcher, and lecturer on topics related to adult and pediatric HIV. She received an M.S. in nutrition and an M.P.H. in Population and Family Health from Columbia University in 1995, and performed her undergraduate studies at the University of Connecticut.

Benjamin N. Hamlin, B.A., research assistant at the Institute of Medicine, received a bachelors degree in biology from the College of Wooster in 1993 and a degree in health sciences from the University of Akron in 1996. He then worked as a surgeon's assistant in the fields of vascular, thoracic, and general surgery for several years before joining the National Academies in 2000. As a research assistant for the Division on Earth and Life Studies at the National Academies, Mr. Hamlin worked with the Board on Radiation Effects Research on projects studying the health effects of ionizing and nonionizing radiation on the human body. In addition to this study, his work at the Institute of Medicine has included the reports *Testosterone and Aging: Clinical Research Directions, Review of NASA's Longitudinal Study of Astronaut Health, Health Literacy: A Prescription to End Confusion,* and *NIH Extramural Center Programs: Criteria for Initiation and Evaluation.* He is currently pursuing graduate work in the sociomedical sciences. He is also involved with the U.S. Bangladesh Advisory Council, an organization that promotes governmental cooperation between the United States and Bangladesh on matters of trade and health care.

Judith L. Estep is senior project assistant for the Board on Health Sciences Policy and the Board on Neuroscience and Behavioral Health. She recently completed work on a project that produced the report *Testosterone and Aging: Clinical Research Directions.* Since coming to the National Academies in 1986 she has provided administrative support for more than 30 published reports. Previously, she worked in the Public Relations Office at The George Washington University Medical Center and with the Department of Social Work.

Index

A

AAMC, *see* Association of American Medical Colleges
Accidents and injuries, 65
   see also Violence
Accreditation, 7, 20, 133
   curricular database, 7
   Curriculum Management and Information Tool (CurrMIT), 26
   Liaison Committee on Medical Education (LCME), 7, 20, 26, 27-31, 50, 121
Aging population, *ix*, 3-4, 17
AIDS, *see* HIV infections
Alcohol use and abuse, 2, 59, 64, 77, 78
Alternative medicine, *see* Complementary and alternative medicine
American Association of Colleges of Osteopathic Medicine, 7, 50
Assessment methodologies
   see also Tests and testing; U.S. Medical Licensing Examination
   committee study at hand, methodology, *x*, 1, 5, 9, 27-28
   Curriculum Management and Information Tool (CurrMIT), 6, 7, 26-31, 51
   databases covering, 1, 7, 21, 26-27, 31-32, 51
   faculty development, 93
   faculty qualifications, 12, 13, 20, 92

formal curriculum change process
      evaluation, 95-96
      needs assessment, 94
   for integrated course content, 22
   medical students' understanding of behavioral/social science, 11, 97-98
   specific university curricula, 37
Association of American Medical Colleges (AAMC), 6, 7, 9, 55, 121
   database of curricula, 26, 31, 50-51
Attitudes and beliefs
   see also Depression and anxiety; Stress, psychosocial
   culture-based, 62-63, 69
   faculty, 49, 89, 93
   patients, 125
   physicians, 8, 10, 16, 23-24, 53, 66-67, 69-70, 125-126
      cultural bias, 62-63, 69
      financial incentives, 85-86
      health policy and economics, 84
      toward pain, 60-61
   "soft" behavioral/social sciences, 89
   student satisfaction with curricula content, 30, 32, 95
Awards
   career development awards programs, 12, 87-88, 91-94
   curriculum development awards, 2, 12, 91, 96-97

B

Barriers to curricular change, *see* Policy issues, barriers to curricular change
Behavioral risk factors, 2, 3, 4, 8, 15-16, 23, 53, 59-60, 63-67, 124-125, 128-129
  see also Nutrition; Stress, psychosocial
  accidents and injuries, 65
  alcohol use and abuse, 2, 59, 64, 77, 78
  biopsychosocial model omits, 17, 23
  diet, 28
  economic incentives affecting, 85
  elderly persons, *ix*, 3-4, 17
  sexual behavior, 48, 59-60, 64-65
  smoking, 2, 15, 50, 63, 77
  as topic to be included in curricula, 1, 10, 11, 55, 56, 58, 63-67
  violence, general, 65

C

CAM, *see* Complementary and alternative medicine
Canada, 26
Career development programs, 2, 12, 87-94, 133
Carnegie Foundation, 21
Chronic conditions, 2, 4, 10, 15, 56, 58, 59, 63, 64, 65, 67, 73
  pain, 61
Communication skills, 4, 8, 23, 24, 29, 53, 128
  see also Physician–patient interactions
  collegial communications, 77
  committee curricular recommendations, 56, 74-76, 130
  counseling, 8, 23, 42, 54, 76, 77
  cultural competence, 56, 80-81, 126
  decision making and, 8, 53, 76, 78
  LCME Hot Topics, 28, 29-31
  role modeling, 25-26, 27
    mentoring, 91, 93
  specific university curricula, 34, 38, 42, 46
Community health, 127
  committee curricular recommendations, 56, 73-74, 130
  LCME Hot Topics, 28, 29, 30
  specific university curricula, 34, 38-40, 42, 44, 46
Complementary and alternative medicine (CAM), 10, 56, 79, 81-82

Continuing medical education, 8, 41, 53, 126
  see also Faculty development
  graduate medical education, *x*, 8, 53
Cost and cost-effectiveness, 3
  as topic to be included in curricula, 10, 83, 85-86
Counseling by physicians, 8, 23, 42, 54, 76, 77
Cultural factors, *see* Sociocultural factors
Curriculum development awards, 2, 12, 91, 96-97
Curriculum Management and Information Tool (CurrMIT), 6, 7, 26-31, 51

D

Databases
  assessment methodologies, 1, 7, 21, 26-27, 31-32, 51
  committee recommendations, 50-51
  curricular content, 1, 6, 7, 20-21, 26, 31, 50-51
  Curriculum Management and Information Tool (CurrMIT), 6, 7, 26-31, 51
  standards for, 6-7, 26, 50
Decision making
  clinical epidemiology, 28-29
  informed consent, 31
  patient-centered care, 16, 35, 41, 53, 76, 78
  patient–physician communication and, 8, 53, 76, 78
Demographic factors, 3-4, 17
  see also Sociocultural factors
  aging population, *ix*, 3-4, 17
  diversity of U.S. population, *ix*, 4, 10, 11, 17-18, 126
    committee curricular recommendations, 10, 11, 56, 57, 58, 68, 69, 72, 79-82, 130
    LCME Hot Topics, 28, 29, 30
    specific university curricula, 34, 36-37, 38, 43, 46
Demonstration projects, 13
Depression and anxiety, 25-26, 59, 60, 61, 62, 67, 71, 76
Diseases and disorders, 60
  see also Behavioral risk factors; End-of-life care; Pain management; Palliative care; Stress, psychosocial
  chronic, 2, 4, 10, 15, 56, 59, 64, 65, 73
  chronic stress, 58, 59, 60, 61, 63
Drug abuse, *see* Substance abuse

E

Economic factors, 1
  see also Awards; Cost and cost-
      effectiveness; Health policy and
      economics
  biopsychosocial model omits, 17
  funding changes, impacts on curricula, 13
  funding for curriculum development, 12-13,
      87, 88, 89, 90
    curriculum demonstration projects, 13,
        97
    curriculum development awards, 2, 12,
        91, 96-97
    faculty, career development awards
        programs, 12, 87-88, 91-94
    faculty development, general 93, 96
    formal curriculum change process, 95,
        96
  funding for teaching and assessment skills,
      88
  health insurance, lack of, 84, 128-129
  inequalities, impact on care, 56, 79-80, 86,
      126-127, 129
  as topic to be included in curricula, 1
    committee recommendations, 10, 11-13,
        56, 57, 83-86, 130, 131
    LCME Hot Topic, 28, 29
    specific university curricula, 35, 39, 43,
        47
Elderly persons, *ix*, 3-4, 17
End-of-life care
  see also Palliative care
  committee curricular recommendations, 77,
      130
  LCME Hot Topics, 28, 29, 30
  specific university curricula, 35, 38, 43, 46
Epidemiology, 130
  LCME Hot Topics, 28, 29, 30
  specific university curricula, 35, 38, 43, 46,
      47
Ethics
  committee curricular recommendations, 4,
      10, 24-25, 56, 68-69
  financial incentives, response to, 85-86
  informed consent, 31
  LCME Hot Topic, 28, 29-31
  specific university curricula, 34, 43, 44
Ethnic groups, *see* Minority groups
Exercise, *see* Physical activity/inactivity

F

Faculty cooperation/resistance, *x*, 12, 49, 50,
      54, 87, 89
  attitudes toward behavioral/social sciences,
      89
Faculty development, 49, 87-94, 132
  assessment techniques, 93
  career development programs, 2, 12, 87-88,
      91-94
  continuing medical education, 92-94
  leadership, 5, 12, 87-88, 89, 90, 91-92, 94-
      95, 132
    career development awards programs, 2,
        12, 87-88, 91-94
    mentoring, 91, 93
  teaching and assessment skills, funding, 88,
      89-90
Faculty qualifications, 12, 13, 20, 22, 89, 92
Family medicine, 62-63
  committee curricular recommendations, 58,
      130
  domestic violence, 35, 38, 43, 47, 127, 130
  specific university curricula, 35, 38-40, 42,
      43, 47, 48
Foreign countries, *see* International
      perspectives
Funding
  changes, impacts on curricula, 13
  curriculum development, 12-13, 87, 88, 89,
      90
    awards, 2, 12, 91, 96-97
    career development awards programs,
        12, 87-88, 91-94
    demonstration projects, 13, 97
    faculty development, general, 93, 96
    formal curriculum change process, 95,
        96
  teaching and assessment skills, 88

G

Genetics, 23, 58, 60, 67, 124
Graduate medical education, *x*, 8, 53

H

Health insurance, lack of, 84, 128-129

Health policy and economics, 128-129
  see also Cost and cost-effectiveness;
      Economic factors; Funding
  biopsychosocial model omits, 17
  committee study, charge, *ix-x*, 5, 19-20
  committee study methodology, *x*, 131
  health insurance, 84, 128, 129
  inequalities, 56, 79-80, 86, 126-127, 129
  as topic to be included in curricula, 1
      committee recommendations, 10, 11-13,
          56, 57, 83-86, 130, 131
      LCME Hot Topic, 28, 29
      specific university curricula, 35, 39, 43,
          47
Health Resources and Services Administration,
      96
Historical perspectives, 20, 21-22, 24
  aging population, *ix*, 3
  behavioral risk factors, 15
  integrated curriculum, 20, 21-22, 33
  life-cycle theories, 60
  variations in care, 86
HIV infections, 59-60
Human development/life cycle, 60, 124-125,
      131
  see also End-of-life care
  LCME Hot Topic, 28, 29, 39
  specific university curricula, 35, 43, 47

I

Injuries, *see* Accidents and injuries
Insurance, *see* Health insurance, lack of
International perspectives, 5
  Canada, 26
  United Kingdom, 86

L

Leadership, 5, 12, 87-88, 89, 90, 91-92, 94-95,
      132
  career development awards programs, 2, 12,
      87-88, 91-94
  mentoring, 91, 93
  role modeling, 25-26, 27
Liaison Committee on Medical Education
      (LCME), 7, 20, 28, 50, 121
  Hot Topics, 27-31
  standards for curricula integration, 26

M

Mentoring, 91, 93
  role modeling, 25-26, 27
Mind–body interactions, 2, 3, 16, 124, 125
  see also Stress, psychosocial
  somatization, 10, 23, 24, 56, 58, 61-62, 120
  as topic to be included in curricula, *x*, 1, 5,
      10, 11, 55, 56, 57, 58
Minority groups
  diversity of U.S. population, *ix*, 4, 10, 11,
      17-18, 126
      committee curricular recommendations,
          10, 11, 56, 57, 58, 68, 69, 72, 79-82,
          130
      LCME Hot Topics, 28, 29, 30
      specific university curricula, 34, 36-37,
          38, 43, 46
  pain, perceptions of, 61
Models and modeling
  behavioral change, 65-66
  biomedical, 17
  biopsychosocial, 6, 12, 16-17, 23, 41
  career development awards program, 2, 12,
      87-88
  chronic care, 73
  combined biomedical/biopsychosocial, 12,
      16, 17
  formal curriculum change process, 94-96
  life-cycle theories, 60
  pain, 60-61

N

National Board of Medical Examiners (NMBE),
      2, 88, 97, 98
  faculty development, 93
  U.S. Medical Licensing Examination, 1, 13,
      88
National Heart, Lung, and Blood Institute, 96
National Institutes of Health
  career development awards programs, 2, 12,
      92
  curriculum development awards programs,
      96-97
  database covering behavioral/social science
      curricula, 7, 51
  demonstration projects, 13
Nutrition, 59
  LCME Hot Topics, 28, 29, 30
  specific university curricula, 44

O

Ohio State University, 34-35, 94-95
Organizational factors
   see also Health policy and economics; Time
     factors; *terms beginning* "Faculty..."
   collegial communications, 77
   committee curricular recommendations, 72-
     73, 83
   formal curriculum change process, 94-96
   leadership, 5, 12, 87-88, 89, 90, 91-92, 94-
     95, 132
      career development awards programs, 2,
       12, 87-88, 91-94
      mentoring, 91, 93

P

Pain management, 3-4, 10, 17, 60-61, 125
   see also End-of-life care
   committee curricular recommendations, 58,
     131
   LCME Hot Topics, 28, 29, 30
   specific university curricula, 35, 39, 44, 47
Palliative care, 131
   see also End-of-life care
   LCME Hot Topics, 28, 29, 30
   specific university curricula, 35, 40, 44, 47
Patient behavior, 63-67
   see also Behavioral risk factors
   as topic to be included in curricula, 1, 10,
     11, 55, 56, 57
Patient health education
   LCME Hot Topics, 28, 29
   specific university curricula, 35, 40, 44, 47
Physical activity/inactivity, 59, 64
Physician–patient interactions, 1, 7, 8, 53-54
   see also Communication skills; Counseling
     by physicians
   attitudes of physician, 8, 10, 16, 23-24, 53,
     66-67, 69-70, 125-126
     cultural bias, 62-63, 69
     toward pain, 60-61
   cultural competence, 56, 80-81, 126
   decision making, 8, 53, 76, 78
   patient-centered care, 16, 35, 41, 53, 76, 78
   problematic patients, 77, 78-79, 128
   somatization, 61-62
   as topic to be included in curricula, *x*, 1, 10,
     11, 56, 57, 74-79

Physician role and behavior, 127, 128
   attitudes, 8, 10, 16, 23-24, 53, 66-67, 69-70,
     125-126
     financial incentives, 85-86
     health policy and economics, 84
   collegial communications, 77
   financial incentives, responses to, 85-86
   medical ethics, 4, 10, 29
   as topic to be included in curricula, *x*, 1, 5,
     10, 11, 56, 57, 68-74, 77
   well-being, 10, 11, 23, 56, 70-71
Policy issues, barriers to curricular change, 87-
   98
   see also Strategies for curriculum change
   committee recommendations, 11-13, 50-51,
     54
   committee study, charge, *ix-x*, 5, 19-20
   committee study methodology, *x*
   complexity of integrated curricula,
     24-25
   databases inadequate, 1, 20, 25-28, 31-32,
     50-51, 90
   faculty cooperation/resistance, *x*, 12, 49, 50,
     54, 87
     attitudes toward behavioral/social
      sciences, 89
   standardization lacking, 6-7, 26, 50, 88
Policy issues, general, *ix*, 1
   see also Economic factors; Health policy
     and economics; Leadership;
     Strategies for curriculum change
   as topic to be included in curricula, *x*, 1, 5,
     10, 11
Population-based medicine, 132
   LCME Hot Topics, 28, 29, 30
   specific university curricula, 35, 40,
     44, 48
Postgraduate education, *see* Graduate medical
   education
Pre-med education, *see* Undergraduate
   education
Preventive medicine and health maintenance,
   132
   see also Behavioral risk factors
   LCME Hot Topics, 28, 29, 30
   specific university curricula, 35, 40, 42, 44,
     48
Problem-based learning, 35, 38-49, 89-90, 130-
   132

Q

Qualifications, faculty, 12, 13, 20, 92
Quality of care, 130
    inequalities, 56, 79-80, 86, 126-127, 129
    LCME Hot Topics, 28, 29, 30
    specific university curricula, 35, 39, 43, 47
Quality of life, 3-4, 17, 85
    end-of-life care
    pain management
    palliative care

R

Research methodology
    see also Databases; Models and modeling
    behavioral and social sciences defined, 5
    committee study at hand, charge, *ix-x*, 1, 4-
        5, 18, 20, 52, 87
    committee study at hand, methodology, *x*, 1,
        5, 9, 27-33, 54-55, 88-89, 119-133
    modified Delphi process, 9, 55, 119,
        121-123
    Curriculum Management and Information
        Tool (CurrMIT), 6, 7, 26-31, 51
Role modeling, 25-26, 27
    mentoring, 91, 93

S

Sexuality and sexual behavior, 59-60, 64-65
    specific university curricula, 48
Small-group teaching methods, 21, 24, 27, 38-
    49 (passim), 89-90, 95, 130-132
Smoking, 2, 15, 50, 63, 77
Sociocultural factors, *x*, 1, 16, 62-63, 126-127,
    133
    accountability and responsibility, 10, 56, 68,
        72
    alternative medicine, 10
    attitudes of physicians, 23-24
    as cause of disease, 2, 15-16
    complementary and alternative medicine
        (CAM), 10, 56, 79, 81-82
    cultural competence, 56, 80-81, 126
    current curricular situation, 29
    diversity of U.S. population, *ix*, 4, 10, 11,
        17-18, 126
        committee curricular recommendations,
            10, 11, 56, 57, 58, 68, 69, 72, 79-82,
            130

LCME Hot Topics, 28, 29, 30
    specific university curricula, 34, 36-37,
        38, 43, 46
    inequalities, 56, 79-80, 126-127, 129
    pain, 61
    substance abuse as curricular topic, 23, 77,
        78, 132
Somatization, 10, 23, 24, 56, 58, 61-62, 120
Standardization
    curricular databases, 6-7, 26, 50
    teaching methods, 26
    U.S. Medical Licensing Examination, 1, 13,
        88
Strategies for curriculum change, 87-98
    see also Awards; Faculty development;
        Leadership; Organizational factors;
        Standardization
    committee recommendations, 11-13, 50, 87
    committee study, charge, *ix-x*, 5, 19-20
Stress, psychosocial, 2-3, 56, 58-59, 60, 61, 66-
    67
    see also Pain management; Violence
    chronic, 58, 59, 60, 61, 63
    depression and anxiety, 25-26, 59, 60, 61,
        62, 67, 71, 76
    immune system effects, 58-59
    on patients, *ix*, 23
    physician well-being, *ix*, 10, 11, 23, 56, 70-
        71
    somatization, 10, 23, 24, 56, 58, 61-62, 120
Substance abuse, 34
    see also Alcohol use and abuse
    biopsychosocial models, 23
    committee curricular recommendations, 23,
        77, 78, 132
    LCME Hot Topics, 28, 29, 30
    specific university curricula, 23, 35, 40, 44,
        48

T

Teaching methods
    career development programs, 91-92, 93
    communication skills, 24, 25
    databases covering, 7, 21, 27, 51
    existing information inadequate, 1, 20, 25-
        26
    faculty development, 89, 94
    faculty qualifications, 12, 13, 20, 22, 89, 92
    formal curriculum change process, 94, 96
    historical perspectives, 21

integration of behavior and social sciences
    into curricula, 33, 36-37
problem-based learning, 35, 38-49, 89-90,
    130-132
role modeling, 25-26, 27
    mentoring, 91, 93
small-group, 21, 24, 27, 38-49 (passim), 89-
    90, 95, 130-132
specific university curricula, 34-49
Tests and testing
    see also Assessment methodologies; U.S.
        Medical Licensing Examination
    faculty development, 93
    formal curriculum change process, 95
    medical students' understanding of
        behavioral/social science, 11, 97-98
Theoretical models, *see* Models and modeling
Time factors
    behavioral/social sciences curricula
        hours taught, 5-6, 26, 28, 29, 31, 32, 34,
            50
        timing of integration, 8-9, 11, 29, 31,
            32, 34-49 (passim), 130-132

    formal curriculum change process, 95-96
    other disciplinary curricula, hours taught, 9
Tobacco use, *see* Smoking

U

Undergraduate education, *x*, 7-8, 53, 123
United Kingdom, 86
University of California, San Francisco, 32, 36-
    40, 93
University of North Carolina, 23, 45-49, 98
University of Rochester, 24-24, 32, 41-45
U.S. Medical Licensing Examination, 1, 13, 88,
    97-98

V

Violence, 65
    domestic, 35, 38, 43, 47, 127, 130